Taping Techniques

Liverpool University Hospital

For Butterworth-Heinemann

Senior Commissioning Editor: Heidi Harrison
Development Editor: Robert Edwards
Project Manager: Joannah Duncan
Design: George Ajayi

Taping Techniques
Principles and Practice

SECOND EDITION

Edited by

Rose Macdonald BA FCSP

Consultant in Sports Physiotherapy, Former Director of the Sports Injury Centre, Crystal Palace National Sports Centre, London, UK

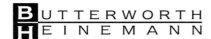

BUTTERWORTH
HEINEMANN

EDINBURGH LONDON NEW YORK OXFORD PHILADELPHIA ST LOUIS SYDNEY TORONTO 2004

BUTTERWORTH-HEINEMANN
An imprint of Elsevier Limited

© Reed Educational and Professional Publishing Ltd 1994
© 2004, Elsevier Limited. All rights reserved.

First edition 1994
Second edition 2004
   Reprinted 2005, 2006, 2007, 2008

ISBN: 978 0 7506 4150 0

British Library Cataloguing in Publication Data
A catalogue record for this book is available from the British Library

Library of Congress Cataloguing in Publication Data
A catalogue record for this book is available from the Library of Congress

Note
Medical knowledge is constantly changing. Standard safety precautions must be followed, but as new research and clinical experience broaden our knowledge, changes in treatment and drug therapy may become necessary or appropriate. Readers are advised to check the most current product information provided by the manufacturer of each drug to be administered to verify there commended dose, the method and duration of administration, and contraindications. It is the responsibility of the practitioner, relying on experience and knowledge of the patient, to determine dosages and the best treatment for each individual patient. Neither the Publisher nor the authors assumes any liability for any injury and/or damage to persons or property arising from this publication.

The Publisher

Contents

Contributors ix

Preface xi

Acknowledgements xiii

PART 1   1

1. Introduction 3
2. Taping literature update 9
3. Taping for pain relief 15
4. Foot types, mechanics and therapy 29

PART 2   59

5. Foot 61

    Turf toe strap 62
    J. O'Neill

    Great toe taping 64
    K.E. Wright

    Hallux valgus 66
    R. Macdonald

    Foot support 68
    G. Lapenskie

    Antipronation taping 70
    A. Hughes

    Plantar fasciitis support 72
    R. Macdonald

    Plantar fasciitis taping 74
    K.E. Wright

    Medial arch support 76
    R. Macdonald

    Cuboid subluxation in dancers 78
    R. Macdonald

    Heel pain 80
    W.A. Hing and D.A. Reid

    Ligament and tendon support 82
    G. Lapenskie

    Calcaneal motion control 84
    G. Lapenskie

6. Ankle and leg 87

    Acute ankle sprain – field wrap 88
    R. Macdonald

    Acute ankle sprain 90
    W.A. Hing and D. A. Reid

    Inferior tibiofibular joint 92
    W.A. Hing and D.A. Reid

    Achilles tendinopathy 94
    W.A. Hing and D.A. Reid

    Ankle dorsiflexion and rear foot motion control 96
    G. Lapenskie

    Achilles tendon support – simple self-application 98
    R. Macdonald

    Achilles tendon support – two methods 100
    O. Rouillon

    Preventive taping for injuries to the lateral aspect of the ankle joint 104
    D. Reese

    Closed basketweave taping for the ankle 108
    R. Macdonald

    Heel locks for closed basketweave 110
    R. Macdonald

    Superior tibiofibular joint 112
    W.A. Hing and D.A. Reid

7. Knee 115

    General knee and/or patellofemoral pain 116
    W.A. Hing and D.A. Reid

    Patellar tendinosis 118
    W.A. Hing and D.A. Reid

    Knee support 120
    G. Lapenskie

Unload the fat pad   122
J. McConnell

Knee support – Crystal Palace
wrap   124
R. Macdonald

Knee support: alternative method –
diamond wrap   126
R. Macdonald

Sprain of the lateral collateral
ligament   128
O. Rouillon

Knee variation to reinforce the
previous basic tape job   130
O. Rouillon

Anterior cruciate taping   132
K.E. Wright

Continuous figure-of-eight wrap for
the knee   134
K.E. Wright

Unstable knee   136
A. DeBruyne

8. Lumbar spine   141

Lumbar spine taping   142
W.A. Hing and D.A. Reid

Frontal plane pelvic stability   144
A. Hughes

Sacroiliac joint   146
W.A. Hing and D.A. Reid

Chronic low-back and leg pain   148
J. McConnell

9. Thoracic spine   151

Thoracic spine taping   152
W.A. Hing and D.A. Reid

Thoracic spine unload   154
D. Kneeshaw

Winging scapulae   156
D. Kneeshaw

Scapular control – Watson's strap   158
D. Kneeshaw

Scapular retraction   160
D. Kneeshaw

10. Shoulder girdle   161

Subluxation of acromioclavicular
joint   162
W.A. Hing and D.A. Reid

Acromioclavicular joint strap   164
D. Kneeshaw

Acromioclavicular joint taping   166
A. Hughes

Acromioclavicular taping for sport
using stretch tape   170
O. Rouillon

Anterior instability – Rigney's
strap   174
D. Kneeshaw

Relocation of the humeral head   176
J. McConnell

Impingement syndrome (Allingham's
strap)   178
D. Kneeshaw

Multidirectional instability   180
J. McConnell

Overactive upper trapezius   182
D. Kneeshaw

11. Elbow, wrist and hand   183

Tennis elbow (lateral epicondylosis)   184
W.A. Hing and D.A. Reid

Simple epicondylitis technique   186
R. Macdonald

Elbow hyperextension sprain   188
R. Macdonald

Prophylactic wrist taping   190
D. Reese

Wrist taping   192
K.E. Wright

Wrist taping   194
R. Macdonald

Inferior radioulnar joint taping   196
W.A. Hing and D.A. Reid

Contusion to the hand   198
K.E. Wright

Palm protective taping (the Russell
web)   200
C. Armstrong

Protection of the metacarpophalangeal joints
for boxers   204
R. Macdonald

12. Fingers and thumb   207

Sprained fingers – buddy system   208
R. Macdonald

Single-finger taping   210
J.O'Neill

Finger joint support   212
R. Macdonald

Climber's finger injury   214
R. Macdonald

Prophylactic thumb taping   216
D. Reese

Simple thumb check–rein figure–of–eight
method   220
R. Macdonald

Thumb spica taping   222
K.E. Wright

13. Stretch tape – many use   225
     R. Macdonald

14. Spicas and triangular bandages   229
     R. Macdonald

Glossary   235

Index   237

Contributors

Chuck Armstrong MScPT MEd
*Armstrong's Physiotherapy Clinic,
Saskatoon, Canada*

Michael J Callaghan PhD MPhil MCSP SRP
*Centre for Rehabilitation Science,
Manchester Royal Infirmary,
Manchester, UK*

Andre DeBruyne MD
Hasselt, Belgium

Wayne Hing MSc(Hons) ADP(OMt) DipMT DipPhys
*School of Physiotherapy, Auckland University of
Technology, Auckland, New Zealand*

Andrew Hughes BAppSc(Phty) MAPA FASMF
*Sports Focus Physiotherapy, Liverpool,
New South Wales, Australia*

David Kneeshaw BAppSc(Phty) MAPA
*Balmain Physiotherapy and Sports, Injury Centre,
Balmain, New South Wales, Australia
(Currently living in the UK)*

Gary Lapenskie BSc(PE) BSc(PT) MA(PE)
*Faculty of Kinesiology, University of Western
Ontario, London, Ontario, Canada*

Rose Macdonald BA FCSP MCPA SRP
*Consultant in Sports Physiotherapy,
London, UK*

Peter Madigan SRCh BEd FCPod(S)
*Division of Podiatry, Faculty of Health,
Glasgow Caledonian University, Glasgow, UK*

Jenny McConnell BAppSci(Phty) GraddipManTher
MBiomedEng
*McConnell & Clements Physiotherapy,
Mosman, New South Wales, Australia*

Susanna R Nickson MPhil BSc(Hons) FCPod(Surg) SRCh
*Podiatry Department, Cross Street Clinic,
Burton on Trent, Staffordshire, UK*

Jeff O'Neill MS ATC
Miami, Florida, USA

Dale Reese BSc
*Medicinskt Centrum Norrköping,
Norrköping, Sweden*

Duncan A Reid BSc DipPhys DipMT PGD(Manips) MNZCP
*School of Physiotherapy, Auckland University of
Technology, Auckland, New Zealand*

Olivier Rouillon MD
Ormesson-sur-mer, France

Kenneth E Wright DA ATC MHSc PGD(ManipPhys)
DipMT DipPhys BSc
*Department of Health Sciences,
University of Alabama,
Tuscaloosa, Alabama, USA*

Preface

In this second edition of *Taping Techniques*, many of the original 'old favourites' are included, as basic techniques are fundamental to the practice of good taping. New contributors from Australia, New Zealand and Europe share their expertise, bringing an abundance of new techniques and updated literature to the volume.

A new chapter explaining the theory and principles behind unloading painful structures and stabilization techniques is included for those who are not familiar with this type of taping. Other new techniques include proprioceptive taping from Australia, Mulligan taping from New Zealand, and new techniques from the USA and Europe.

Functional taping is now recognized as a skill which is essential for those involved in the treatment and rehabilitation of sports injuries. Taping is widely used, not only for sports injuries but for many other conditions, such as muscle imbalances, unstable joints and neural control. Proprioceptive taping is playing a greater role in the treatment of some conditions; it is a useful tool for reminding the patient, by skin drag, not to perform a specific movement which is contrary to the treatment of the condition. During treatment and rehabilitation, taping aids the healing process by supporting and protecting the injured structures from further injury or stress.

Taping reduces the need for prolonged treatment and reduces time off sport or work for the patient. Many techniques are useful for the non-sports-player and may be used by the practitioner in general practice or in the hospital environment.

Sports medicine leans towards early mobilization through functional therapy, and total immobilization in plaster casts is less common now. Removable cast bracing is used to enable therapy to continue throughout the postoperative phase.

Tape becomes a 'flexible cast' which aids in the prevention of athletic injuries and rests the injured parts in order to aid healing. Flexible tape casts limit range of motion and may be used in many sports where rigid supports are not allowed.

Since taping is essentially practical, new techniques are constantly being developed, not only to prevent injuries but also to allow patients to return to work or sport more quickly by using tape effectively. Once the basic techniques are mastered, it is then up to practitioners to modify, change and develop new techniques themselves, always adhering to the basic taping principles.

To aid in the development of new techniques, this book is full of new ideas, which may be used as indicated or modified to suit the situation. The book brings an abundance of new international techniques to the reader, many of which are simple to apply and are very effective.

Podiatry is now playing a greater role in sports medicine; therefore, the chapter on podiatry has been considerably updated to include current trends.

Some 'quickies' or 'many uses' for one strip of tape are also included. Common sense and an imaginative mind can create a simple temporary support. Bandaging now seems to be a thing of the past and is not taught to undergraduate students. Therefore, a short section on spica (figure-of-eight) bandaging is included. On some occasions a bandage is more appropriate than tape. Spicas are mainly used to hold protective pads or devices in place during training or competition. Finally, a section called 'Spicas and Triangular Bandages' is included for quick reference.

Rose Macdonald, 2004

Acknowledgements

First, I wish to thank all the contributors for sharing their proven techniques and for their cooperation and patience.

I should also like to thank Butterworth-Heinemann for inviting me to compile and edit this new edition of *Taping Techniques*. I am grateful to their production team for designing the layout of the book in such a way that the text and diagrams are easy to follow and understand at a glance.

St John Ambulance have kindly allowed their diagrams to be used as an 'aide memoire'.

PART 1

PART CONTENTS

1. Introduction   3
2. Taping literature update   9
3. Taping for pain relief   15
4. Foot types, mechanics and therapy   29

Chapter 1

Introduction

R. Macdonald

CHAPTER CONTENTS

Role of taping   3
Storage   7

Taping terms   7

The application of tape to injured soft tissues and joints provides support and protection for these structures and minimizes pain and swelling in the acute stage. Tape should reinforce the normal supportive structures in their relaxed position and protect the injured tissues from further damage. Many different techniques are used for injury prevention, treatment, rehabilitation, proprioception and sport.

Various techniques are illustrated in this manual, together with different philosophies expressed by the contributors – many of whom are eminent physical therapists in their respective countries.

ROLE OF TAPING

Initially, tape is applied to protect the injured structure, during the treatment and rehabilitation programme:

- to hold dressings and pads in place
- to compress recent injury, thus reducing bleeding and swelling
- to protect from further injury by supporting ligaments, tendons and muscles
- to limit unwanted joint movement
- to allow optimal healing without stressing the injured structures
- to protect and support the injured structure in a functional position during the exercise, strengthening and proprioceptive programme.

It must be clearly understood that taping is not a substitute for treatment and rehabilitation, but is an adjunct to the total-injury-care programme.

Tape and wrapping products

Good-quality tape should adhere readily and maintain adhesion despite perspiration and activity.

Stretch (elastic) adhesive tape conforms to the contours of the body, allowing for normal tissue expansion and is used for the following:

- to compress and support soft tissue
- to provide anchors around muscle, thus allowing for expansion
- to hold protective pads in place.

Stretch tape will not give mechanical support to ligaments, but may be used in conjunction with rigid tape to give added support. Stretch tape is not normally tearable and must be cut with scissors, but there are now available very light-weight stretch tapes which may be torn by hand. Stretch tape is available in a variety of widths, from 1.25 to 10 cm, and sometimes even wider. Stretch tape may have:

- one-way stretch, in length or width
- two-way stretch, in length and width.

Stretch tape tends to roll back on itself at the cut ends, therefore it is wise to allow the last couple of centimetres to recoil before sticking it down.

Non-stretch adhesive tape has a non-yielding cloth backing and is used for the following:

- to support inert structures, e.g. ligaments, joint capsule
- to limit joint movement
- to act prophylactically
- to secure the ends of stretch tape
- to reinforce stretch tape
- to enhance proprioception.

Non-stretch tape should be torn by hand to maintain tension during application. It is important to be able to tear the tape from various positions – practice will help to attain a high level of efficiency.

Technique

Tear the tape close to the roll, keeping it taut. Hold the tape with the thumb and index fingers close together. Rip the tape quickly in scissors fashion. Practise tearing a strip of tape into very small pieces in both directions, lengthwise and crossways.

Hypoallergenic tapes are available, offering an alternative to conventional zinc oxide adhesive tape, to which some athletes are allergic.

Waterproof tape is also available in many widths.

Cohesive bandages are a useful product and may be used instead of stretch tape. The product sticks to itself and not to the skin, is waterproof and is reusable. These are most useful when applying spica bandages or as a cover-up for any tape procedure.

Return to activity

On return to activity the injured area is still at risk. Reinjury can be prevented by taping the weakened area, with the aim of restricting joint and muscle movement to within safe limits. This allows performance with confidence.

Lax and hypermobile joints may also be supported with adhesive tape in order to reduce the risk of injury during sport.

Taping principles

The application of tape is easy, but if it is not carried out correctly it will be of little value, and may even be detrimental. Therefore knowledge of the basic principles and practical aspects is essential if the full value of the technique is to be attained.

A thorough assessment is necessary before taping any structure. The following questions should be answered:

Notes

If you are considering taping a player on the field, ensure that the use of tape does not contravene the rules of the sport, thus making the player ineligible to participate. *Know the sport.* Is there time allowed for taping on the field? Or do you have to remove the player from the field of play in order to apply tape? You must also consider the event in which the athlete is participating.

- Has the injury been thoroughly assessed?
- How did the injury occur?
- What structures were damaged?
- What tissues need protection and support?
- What movements must be restricted?
- Is the injury acute or chronic?
- Is immobilization necessary at this stage?
- Are you familiar with the anatomy and biomechanics of the parts involved?
- Can you visualize the purpose for which the tape is to be applied?
- Are you familiar with the technique?
- Do you have suitable materials at hand?

Taping guidelines

Prepare the area to be taped.

- Wash, dry and shave the skin in a downward direction.
- Remove oils for better adhesion.
- Cover broken lesions before taping; an electric shaver avoids cutting the skin.
- Check if the athlete is allergic to tape or spray.
- Apply lubricated protective padding to friction and pressure areas.

- Apply adhesive spray for skin protection and better tape adhesion.

- Apply underwrap for sensitive skin.

Tips

If the area is frequently taped, move the anchor point on successive tapings to prevent skin irritation.

Tape application

- Have all the required materials at hand.

- Have the athlete and yourself in a comfortable position, e.g. couch at an optimal working height, to avoid fatigue.

- Apply tape to skin which is at room temperature.

- Have the full attention of the athlete.

- Place the joint in a functional position, with minimum stress on the injured structure.

- Ensure that the ligaments are in the shortened position.

- Use the correct type, width and amount of tape for the procedure.

- Apply strips of tape in a sequential order.

- Overlap successive strips by half to prevent slippage and gapping.

- Apply each strip with a particular purpose in mind.

- Apply tape smoothly and firmly.

- Flow with the shape of the limb.

- Explain the function of the tape to the athlete, and how it should feel.

- On completion, check that the tape is functional and comfortable.

Tips

For acutely angled areas, rip the tape longitudinally into strips. Small strips are easier to conform by lapping them over each other.

The tape should conform with even pressure and must be effective and comfortable. Tape applied directly to the skin gives maximum support.

Avoid

- excessive traction on skin – this may lead to skin breakdown
- gaps and wrinkles – these may cause blisters
- continuous circumferential taping – single strips produce a more uniform pressure

- excessive layers of tape – this may impair circulation and neural transmission
- too tight an application over bony areas – this may cause bone ache.

Tape removal

Never rip tape off, especially from the plantar aspect of the foot. Use a tape cutter or bandage scissors for safe, fast removal. Lubricate the tip with petroleum jelly and slide it parallel to the skin in the natural soft-tissue channels.

Remove the tape carefully by peeling it back on itself, and pushing the skin away from the tape.

Pull the tape carefully along the axis of the limb.

Check the skin for damage and apply lotion to restore skin moisture. Tape should not be left on for more than 24 h, unless using hypoallergenic tape which may be left on longer. Leaving tape on for too long a period may lead to skin breakdown.

STORAGE

Tape with zinc oxide adhesive mass is susceptible to temperature change and should be stored in a cool place. Tape should be left in its original packing until required. Partially used rolls should be kept in an airtight container (e.g. cooler box or plastic box) and not left on shelves. At temperatures over 20°C the adhesive mass becomes sticky, making the tension stronger and thus more difficult to unwind. Non-stretch tape is also more difficult to tear when warm. Hypoallergenic tapes are not susceptible to temperature change.

TAPING TERMS

Anchors: the first strips of tape applied above and below the injury site, and to which subsequent strips are attached. Anchors minimize traction on the skin (skin drag) and are applied without tension.

Support strips and stirrups restrict unwanted sideways movement.

Gibney/horizontal strips add stability to the joint.

Reinforcing strips restrict movement and add tensile strength to strategic areas when applied over stretch tape.

Check reins restrict range of motion.

Lock strips secure the cut end of stretch tape, which tends to roll back on itself, secure check reins in place, and neatly finish the technique when applied over anchors (fill strips).

Heel locks give additional support to the subtalar and ankle joints.

Notes

Use stirrups and Gibney strips alternately, to form a basketweave pattern.

Taping products

Underwrap/prowrap: thin polyurethane foam material used to protect sensitive skin from zinc oxide adhesive mass.

Gauze squares: foam squares, or heel-and-lace pads are used to protect areas which are susceptible to stress and friction.

Padding: felt, foam rubber or other materials for protecting sensitive areas.

Adhesive spray: applied to make skin tacky and thus help underwrap, protective pads or tape adhere more readily.

Dehesive spray: breaks down the adhesive mass and allows tape to be removed easily.

Tape remover: available as spray, solution or wipes to clean adhesive residue from the skin.

Petroleum jelly: applied to lubricate areas of stress and reduce friction and irritation to the soft tissues.

Talcum powder: used to remove adhesive residue where necessary; it also prevents stretch tape from rolling at the edges.

Cohesive bandage: adheres to itself but not to the skin and can be used for light compression or applied over tape to prevent unravelling in water.

Tubular bandage: may be applied over completed tape job to help set the tape and hold it in place.

Elastic bandage/tensor: used for compression and for traditional spicas.

Cloth wrap: used for ankle wraps, triangular bandages, collar and cuff support.

Tape cutter: allows quick and safe removal of tape.

Bandage scissors: flat-ended scissors for safe removal of tape.

Other useful products

A variety of athletic braces and supports for body parts, neoprene/elastic/other sleeves, rubber tubing, extra-long tensor/cohesive bandages for spicas, hot/cold packs, second-skin/blister kit.

Chapter **2**

Taping literature update

M.J. Callaghan

CHAPTER CONTENTS

Introduction   9
Ankle taping   9
Injury prevention   11
Prewrap   11

Taping technique   11
Patellar taping   11
References   12

INTRODUCTION

Taping continues to be an essential part of a physiotherapist's armamentarium in the various stages of rehabilitation after injury. Indeed, many athletes consider taping such an essential part of their sporting preparation that it becomes a ritualistic process, occasionally verging on the superstitious! This should not distract us from continuing to investigate the scientific rationale behind its application from the growing wealth of literature. This chapter deals with the literature concerning both ankle taping and patellar taping.

ANKLE TAPING

The literature on ankle taping is considerable, mainly because ankles are easily studied by X-ray, electromyography, goniometry and kinetic and kinematic analysis. The rationale for ankle taping mainly involves treatment of controlling oedema, mechanical instability and functional instability.

Controlling oedema

After an acute ligament sprain of the ankle, compressive strapping is often recommended and applied to control oedema (McCluskey et al 1976). Very few studies have been published to evaluate the efficacy of taping to achieve limb or joint compression. Viljakka (1986) and Rucinski et al (1991) came to conflicting conclusions as to the effect of bandaging on acute ankle oedema. Further studies using ankle bracing or taping after acute injury include several randomized controlled trials comparing ankle bracing or taping with surgery

(Möller-Larsen et al 1988, Specchiulli et al 1997), partial weight-bearing (Karlsson et al 1996), immobilization (Eiff et al 1994), compression or elasticated bandages (Muwanga et al 1986; O'Hara et al 1992, Leanderson & Wredmark 1995). The evidence from these studies points to short-term improved function and a quicker return to work compared with immobilization or compression bandages and, more importantly, equal long-term efficacy compared with surgery.

Mechanical instability

Preventing extremes of range of movement and reducing the abnormal movement of the ankle is the most obvious role of ankle taping. On normal subjects, tape has been demonstrated to reduce extremes of ankle range of movement after 15 min running over a figure-of-eight course (Laughman et al 1980). On patients with proven mechanical ankle instability, a zinc oxide Gibney basketweave technique significantly decreased the amount of non-weight-bearing talar tilt (Larsen 1984, Vaes et al 1985). It was noted that those patients with the greatest instability received the greatest benefit from the tape. Although taping does seem to improve mechanical instability, it is important to note that the restricting effect is lost after varying periods of exercise. For example, 40% of the effect of taping was lost after 10 min of vigorous general circuit exercises (Rarick et al 1962). Approximately 50% was lost after 15 min of standard vigorous exercises (Frankeny et al 1993); there was a 20% decrease after 20 min stop/start running (Larsen 1984), 37% loosening in total passive range of motion after 20 min of volleyball training (Greene & Hillman 1990), 10–20% restriction loss in all movements except dorsiflexion after 60 min of squash (Myburgh et al 1984) and a 14% loss of inversion restriction after 30 min of exercise (Alt et al 1999).

It is this inability to maintain mechanical stability during exercise that raises fundamental questions and proposes alternative theories behind taping and bracing.

Functional instability

Freeman et al (1965) seem to be amongst the first to describe functional instability as 'a term … to designate the disability to which the patients refer when they say that their foot tends to "give way"'. Although initially ignored, there has been more recent interest in the concept of functional instability of the ankle and the role of taping and bracing to alleviate it. As a result, some authors have investigated the protective role of taping and bracing on the 'proprioception' of the chronically injured ankle (Glick et al 1976, Hamill et al 1986, Karlsson & Andreasson 1992, Jerosch et al 1995, Lentell et al 1995, Robbins et al 1995). Proprioceptive control of the ankle (and thus the effect of taping and bracing) has been measured by a variety of tests, such as peroneal reflex activity (Karlsson & Andreasson 1992, Konradsen & Hojsgaard 1993; Konradsen et al 1993; Feuerbach et al 1994; Ashton-Miller et al 1996; Lohrer et al 1999), joint angle reproduction (Jerosch et al 1995, Lentell et al 1995, Refshauge et al 2000) and movement threshold (Konradsen et al 2000).

INJURY PREVENTION

Epidemiological studies have established the ability of tape and braces to prevent recurrent ankle injury. The most commonly cited study on injury prevention is that of Garrick & Requa (1973), which studied the effect of taping on 2563 basketball players with previous ankle sprains over two successive seasons. They concluded that a zinc oxide stirrup with horseshoe and figure-of-eight technique, in combination with high-top shoe, had a protective influence (6.5 injuries/1000 games) for preventing ankle sprains.

Ankle braces may also lead to a reduction in the incidence and severity of acute ankle sprains in competition (Bahr et al 1994), such as basketball (Sitler et al 1994), men's football (soccer) (Tropp et al 1985, Surve et al 1994), and women's football (Sharpe et al 1997). Although the studies reviewed provide important information regarding efficacy of tape or a brace, criticisms have been made regarding study design, external validity, confounding variables and sample size (Sitler et al 1994). These should also be considered before selecting the appropriate technique or device.

Thus there is some evidence that ankle sprains can be prevented by ankle supports during sports like football (soccer) and basketball, with the reduction in injury greater for those with previous ankle sprain.

PREWRAP

Two studies have looked at the effects of prewrap on taping that should ease the reservations amongst clinicians of the effects of pre-wrap or underwrap on taping. Manfroy et al (1997) used 20 healthy subjects to perform 40 min of exercise and found no statistically significant differences in experimental limitation of inversion moments between ankle taping with and without prewrap. Ricard et al (2000) measured the amount and rate of dynamic ankle inversion using a trapdoor inversion platform apparatus and concluded that applying tape over prewrap was as effective as applying it directly to skin.

TAPING TECHNIQUE

The lack of comparative studies between different taping techniques helps to explain why the choice of tape by athletes and physiotherapists is often governed by personal preference, the experience of the person applying the tape and a general feel as to the correct technique.

Of those few studies, Rarick et al (1962) favoured a basketweave with stirrup and heel-lock technique. Frankeny et al (1993) concluded that the Hinton–Boswell method (in which the ankle is taped in a relaxed plantarflexed position) provided greatest resistance to inversion. Metcalfe et al (1997) compared zinc oxide closed basketweave with heel locks and figure-of-eight, reinforced with moleskin tape to a Swede-O-Universal brace and found no differences between the three methods in terms of talocrural and subtalar range of motion.

PATELLAR TAPING

The investigations into the relationship between mechanical and functional aspects of ankle taping are paralleled over the years by those on patellar taping. It is well known that McConnell (1986) originally described patellar taping as part of a treatment programme for patellofemoral pain syndrome (PFPS) and theorized that this technique could alter patellar position, enhance contraction of the vastus medialis oblique (VMO) muscle, and hence decrease pain.

It is becoming clear from recent literature reviews on this subject (Callaghan 1997, Crossley et al 2000) that studies thus far on patients with PFPS have been inconclusive regarding patellar taping enhancement of VMO contractions and taping realignment of patellar position. Nevertheless, many studies have shown that patellar taping helps decrease pain in patients with PFPS (Bockrath et al 1993, Cerny 1995, Herrington & Payton 1997, Powers et al 1997, Somes et al 1997) and in patellofemoral osteoarthritis (Cushnaghan et al 1995), although the mechanism for this symptomatic improvement remains unknown.

More recently, there has been speculation that there may be a more subtle role for patellar taping in providing sensory feedback and influence on the proprioceptive status and neuromuscular control of the patellofemoral joint. For example, Callaghan et al (2002) showed that a simple application of one 10-cm strip of patellar taping significantly improves the knee proprioceptive status of healthy subjects whose proprioception was graded as 'poor'. At the same time, Baker et al (2002) showed that patients with PFPS had worse proprioception compared to a group of healthy subjects. It is tempting therefore to speculate that patients with patellofemoral pain may have enhanced proprioception after the application of tape, and this may explain the short-term subjective improvement without any firm evidence of patellar alignment or VMO-enhanced contractions.

References

Alt W, Lohrer H, Gollhofer A 1999 Functional properties of adhesive ankle taping: neuromuscular and mechanical effects before and after exercise. Foot and Ankle International 20(4): 238–245

Ashton-Miller J A, Ottaviani R A, Hutchinson C, Wojtys E M 1996 What best protects the inverted weight bearing ankle against further inversion? American Journal of Sports Medicine 24(6): 800–809

Bahr R, Karlsen R, Lian O, Ovrebo R V 1994 Incidence and mechanisms of acute ankle inversion injuries in volleyball. American Journal of Sports Medicine 22(5): 595–600

Baker V, Bennell K, Stillman B et al 2002 Abnormal knee joint position sense in individuals with patellofemoral pain syndrome. Journal of Orthopaedic Research 20: 208–214

Bockrath K, Wooden C, Worrell T W et al 1993 Effects of patellar taping on patellar position and perceived pain. Medicine and Science in Sport and Exercise 25(9): 989–992

Callaghan M J 1997 Patellar taping, the theory versus the evidence: a review. Physical Therapy Reviews 2: 181–183

Callaghan M J, Selfe J, Bagley P, Oldham J A 2002 The effect of patellar taping on knee joint proprioception. Journal of Athletic Training 37(1): 19–24

Cerny K 1995 Vastus medialis oblique/vastus lateralis muscle activity for selected exercises in persons with and without patellofemoral pain syndrome. Physical Therapy 75(8): 672–683

Crossley K, Cowan S M, Bennell K L, McConnell J 2000 Patellar taping: is clinical success supported by scientific evidence? Manual Therapy 5(3): 142–150

Cushnaghan J, McCarthy C, Dieppe P 1995 Taping the patella medially: a new treatment for osteoarthritis of the knee. British Medical Journal 308: 753–755

Eiff M P, Smith A T, Smith G E 1994 Early mobilisation versus immobilisation in the treatment of lateral ankle sprains. American Journal of Sports Medicine 22(1): 83–88

Feuerbach J W, Grabiner M D, Koh T J, Weiker G G 1994 Effect of an ankle orthosis and ankle ligament anesthesia on ankle joint proprioception. American Journal of Sports Medicine 22(2): 223–229

Frankeny J R, Jewett D L, Hanks G A, Sebastianelli W J 1993 A comparison of ankle taping methods. Clinical Journal of Sports Medicine 3: 20–25

Freeman M A R, Dean M R E, Hanham I W F 1965 The etiology and prevention of functional instability of the foot. Journal of Bone and Joint Surgery (Br) 47-B(4): 678–685

Garrick J G, Requa R K 1973 Role of external support in the prevention of ankle sprains. Medicine and Science in Sports 5(3): 200–203

Glick J M, Gordon R M, Nishimoto D 1976 The prevention and treatment of ankle injuries. American Journal of Sports Medicine 4: 136–141

Greene T A, Hillman S K 1990 Comparison of support provided by a semirigid orthosis and adhesive ankle taping before, during and after exercise. American Journal of Sports Medicine 18(5): 498–506

Hamill J, Knutzen K M, Bates B T, Kirkpatrick G 1986 Evaluation of two ankle appliances using ground reaction force data. Journal of Orthopedic and Sports Physical Therapy 7(5): 244–249

Herrington L, Payton C J 1997 Effects of corrective taping of the patella on patients with patellofemoral pain. Physiotherapy 83(11): 566–572

Jerosch J, Hoffstetter I, Bork H, Bischof M 1995 The influence of orthoses on the proprioception of the ankle joint. Knee Surgery, Sports Traumatology, Arthroscopy 3: 39–46

Karlsson J, Andreasson G O 1992 The effect of external ankle support in chronic lateral ankle joint instability. American Journal of Sports Medicine 20(3): 257–261

Karlsson J, Eriksson E, Sward L 1996 Early functional treatment for acute ligament injuries of the ankle joint. Scandinavian Journal of Medicine and Science in Sports 6: 341–345

Konradsen L, Beynnon B D, Renström P A 2000 Techniques for measuring sensorimotor control of the ankle: evaluation of different methods. In: Lephart S M, Fu F H (eds) Proprioception and Neuromuscular Control in Joint Stability, pp. 139–144. Human Kinetics, Champaign, IL

Konradsen L, Hojsgaard C 1993 Pre-heel-strike peroneal muscle activity during walking and running with and without an external ankle support. Scandinavian Journal of Medicine and Science in Sports 3: 99–103

Konradsen L, Ravn J, Sorensen A I 1993 Proprioception at the ankle: the effect of anaesthetic blockade of ligament receptors. Journal of Bone and Joint Surgery (Br) 75-B(3): 433–436

Larsen E 1984 Taping the ankle for chronic instability. Acta Orthopaedica Scandinavica 55: 551–553

Laughman R K, Carr T A, Chao E Y et al 1980 Three dimensional kinematics of the taped ankle before and after exercise. American Journal of Sports Medicine 8(6): 425–431

Leanderson J, Wredmark T 1995 Treatment of acute ankle sprain. Comparison of a semi-rigid ankle brace and compression bandage in 73 patients. Acta Orthopaedica Scandinavica 66(6): 529–531

Lentell G, Baas B, Lopez D et al 1995 The contributions of proprioceptive deficits, muscle function, and anatomic laxity to functional instability of the ankle. Journal of Orthopedic and Sports Physical Therapy 21(4): 206–215

Lohrer H, Alt W, Gollhofer A 1999 Neuromuscular properties and functional aspects of taped ankles. American Journal of Sports Medicine 27(1): 69–75

Manfroy P P, Ashton-Miller J A, Wojtys E M 1997 The effect of exercise, prewrap and athletic tape on the maximal active and passive ankle resistance to ankle inversion. American Journal of Sports Medicine 25(2): 156–163

McCluskey G M, Blackburn T A, Lewis T 1976 A treatment for ankle sprains. American Journal of Sports Medicine 4(4): 158–161

McConnell J 1986 The management of chondromalacia patellae: a long term solution. Australian Journal of Physiotherapy 32(4): 215–223

Metcalfe R C, Schlabach G A, Looney M A, Renehan E J 1997 A comparison of moleskin tape, linen tape and lace up brace on joint restriction and movement performance. Journal of Athletic Training 32(2): 136–140

Möller-Larsen F, Wethelund J O, Jurik A G et al 1988 Comparison of three different treatments for ruptured lateral ankle ligaments. Acta Orthopaedica Scandinavica 59(5): 564–566

Muwanga C L, Quinton D N, Sloan J P et al 1986 A new treatment of stable ligament injuries of the ankle. Injury 17(6): 380–382

Myburgh K H, Vaughan C L, Isaacs S K 1984 The effects of ankle guards and taping on joint motion before, during and after a squash match. American Journal of Sports Medicine 12(6): 441–446

O'Hara J, Valle-Jones J C, Walsh H et al 1992 Controlled trial of an ankle support (Malleotrain) in acute ankle injuries. British Journal of Sports Medicine 26(3): 139–142

Powers C M, Landel R, Sosnick T et al 1997 The effects of patellar taping on stride characteristics and joint motion in subjects with patellofemoral pain. Journal of Orthopedic and Sports Physical Therapy 26(6): 286–291

Rarick G L, Bigley G, Karts R, Malina R M 1962 The measurable support of the ankle joint by conventional methods of taping. Journal of Bone and Joint Surgery (Am) 44-A(6): 1183–1190

Refshauge K M, Kilbreath S L, Raymond J 2000 The effect of recurrent ankle inversion sprain and taping on proprioception at the ankle. Medicine and Science in Sport and Exercise 32(1): 10–15

Ricard M D, Sherwood S M, Schulthies S S, Knight K L 2000 Effects of tape and exercise on dynamic ankle inversion. Journal of Athletic Training 35(1): 31–37

Robbins S, Waked E, Rappel R 1995 Ankle taping improves proprioception before and after exercise in young men. British Journal of Sports Medicine 29(4): 242–247

Rucinski T J, Hooker D N, Prentice W E et al 1991 The effects of intermittent compression on edema in postacute ankle sprains. Journal of Orthopedic and Sports Physical Therapy 14(2): 65–69

Sharpe S R, Knapik J, Jones B 1997 Ankle braces effectively reduce recurrence of ankle sprains in female soccer players. Journal of Athletic Training 32(1): 21–24

Sitler M, Ryan J, Wheeler B et al 1994 The efficacy of a semirigid ankle stabilizer to reduce acute ankle injuries in basketball. American Journal of Sports Medicine 22(4): 454–461

Somes S, Worrell T W, Corey B, Ingersoll C D 1997 Effects of patellar taping on patellar position in the open and closed kinetic chain: a preliminary study. Journal of Sport Rehabilitation 6(4): 299–308

Specchiulli F, Scialpi L, Solarino G et al 1997 Comparison of surgery, cast immobilisation and taping in the treatment of garde III ankle sprains. Journal of Sports Traumatology and Related Research 19(1): 1–6

Surve I, Schwellnus M P, Noakes T, Lombard C 1994 A fivefold reduction in the incidence of recurrent ankle sprains in soccer players using the sport-stirrup orthosis. American Journal of Sports Medicine 22(5): 601–605

Tropp H, Askling C, Gillquist J 1985 Prevention of ankle sprains. American Journal of Sports Medicine 13(4): 259–262

Vaes P, DeBoeck H, Handelberg F, Opdecam P 1985 Comparative radiological study of the influence of ankle joint strapping and taping on ankle stability. Journal of Orthopedic and Sports Physical Therapy 7(3): 110–114

Viljakka T 1986 Mechanics of knee and ankle bandages. Acta Orthopaedica Scandinavica 57: 54–58

Chapter **3**

Taping for pain relief

J. McConnell

CHAPTER CONTENTS

Minimizing the aggravation of inflamed
  tissue – unloading painful structures   16
Effect of tape   17
Patellar taping   18
Case study 1   19
Specific VMO training   20
Unloading neural tissue – a strategy
  for managing chronic low–back and
  leg pain   21

Shoulder taping – repositioning
  or unloading   24
Case study 2   25
Conclusion   26
References   26

Pain is the most frequent complaint of patients presenting for treatment at sports medicine clinics. However, pain is usually not the result of an acute one-off injury but of habitual imbalances in the movement system, which over time cause chronic problems. The management of musculoskeletal symptoms is therefore extremely challenging for the clinician, as symptom reduction alone is not sufficient for a successful treatment outcome, particularly when dealing with athletes who need to be finely tuned for the extraordinary demands placed on their bodies. Often it is difficult for the clinician to determine the cause and origin of the pain as there may be confounding hyper/hypomobility problems of the surrounding soft tissues. One of the greatest challenges for a patient is finding appropriate strategies to stabilize any unstable segments, as success in this area will ensure fewer recurrences and perhaps a higher return of function.

Joint stability requires the interaction of three different subsystems – the passive (the bones, ligaments, fascia and any other non-contractile tissue such as discs and menisci), the active (the muscles acting on the joints) and the neural (central nervous system and nerves controlling the muscles) subsystems (Panjabi 1992a). The most vulnerable area of a joint is known as the neutral zone, where little resistance is offered by the passive structures (Panjabi 1992b). Dysfunction of the passive, active or neural systems will affect the neutral zone and hence the stability of the joint. The size of the neutral zone can be increased by injury and decreased with muscle strengthening. In the spine, for example, stability of a segment can be increased by muscle activity of as little as 1–3% (Cholewicki et al 1997). Uncompensated dysfunction, however, will ultimately cause pathology.

How long will it take before uncompensated movement causes symptoms? The answer to this question is probably best determined by Dye's model of tissue homeostasis of a joint (1996). Dye contends that symptoms will only occur when an individual is no longer operating inside his/her envelope of function, reaching a particular threshold and thereby causing a complex biological cascade of trauma and repair, manifesting clinically as pain and swelling. The threshold varies from individual to individual, depending on the amount and frequency of the loading (Dye 1996, Novacheck 1997). Four factors (anatomic, kinematic, physiological and treatment) are pertinent in determining the size of the envelope of function (Dye 1996, Dye et al 1998). The therapist can have a positive influence on the patient's envelope of function by minimizing the aggravation of the inflamed tissue and can perhaps even increase the patient's threshold of function by improving the control over the mobile segments and the movement of the stiff segments (McConnell 2000).

MINIMIZING THE AGGRAVATION OF INFLAMED TISSUE – UNLOADING PAINFUL STRUCTURES

The concept of minimizing the aggravation of inflamed tissue is certainly central to all interventions in orthopaedics. Clinicians have a number of weapons in their armoury, such as anti-inflammatory medication, topical creams, ice, electrotherapy modalities, acupuncture and tape, to attack pain and reduce inflammation. It is in the chronic state that pain is more difficult to settle and sometimes symptoms seem to be increased by the very treatment that is designed to diminish them. For example, a patient with chronic low-back and leg pain with restricted forward flexion treated in slump to increase range, experiences a marked exacerbation of the symptoms. This patient becomes reluctant to have further treatment for fear of further increases of pain; thus, the range becomes more restricted, further reducing the patient's activity. Another patient, with chronic fat pad irritation, is given straight-leg-raise exercises, only to find the pain worsens, so avoids further treatment and limits activity, which hastens the quadriceps atrophy, resulting in lateral tracking of the patella and further increases in pain.

Key to the success of management of these patients is to unload the inflamed soft tissues to break the endless cycle of increased pain and decreased activity, which allows the clinician to address the patient's poor dynamic control. The principle of unloading is based on the premise that inflamed soft tissue does not respond well to stretch (Gresalmer & McConnell 1998). For example, if a patient presents with a sprained medial collateral ligament, applying a valgus stress to the knee will aggravate the condition, whereas a varus stress will decrease the symptoms. Tape can be used to unload (shorten) the inflamed tissue and perhaps improve joint alignment by providing a constant low load on the soft tissue. It has been widely documented that the length of soft tissues can be increased with sustained stretching (Hooley et al 1980, Herbert 1993). If the tape can be maintained for a prolonged period of time, then this, plus muscle training of the stabilizing muscles actively to change the joint position, be it patellofemoral or glenohumeral, should have a significant effect on the mechanics.

There is some debate as to whether tape can actually change joint position. Most of the research has examined changes in patellar position. Some investigators have found that tape changes patellofemoral (PF) angle and lateral patellar displacement, but congruence angle is not changed (Roberts 1989). Others have concurred, finding no change in congruence angle when the patella is taped, but congruence angle is measured at 45° knee flexion, so subtle changes in patellar position may have occurred before this (Bockrath et al 1993). A recent study of asymptomatic subjects found that medial glide tape was effective in moving the patella medially ($P = 0.003$), but ineffective in maintaining the position after vigorous exercise ($P < 0.001$). But, tape seemed to prevent the lateral shift of the patella that occurred with exercise ($P = 0.016$) (Larsen et al 1995). The issue for a therapist, however, is not whether the tape changes the patellar position on X-ray, but whether the therapist can immediately decrease the patient's symptoms by at least 50%, so the patient can exercise and train in a painfree manner.

EFFECT OF TAPE

The effect of tape on pain, particularly patellofemoral pain, has been fairly well established in the literature (Conway et al 1992, Bockrath et al 1993, Cerny 1995, Powers et al 1997, Gilleard et al 1998). Even in an older age group (mean age 70 years) with tibiofemoral osteoarthritis, taping the patella in a medial direction resulted in a 25% reduction in knee pain (Cushnagan et al 1994). However, the mechanism of the effect is still widely debated.

It has been found that taping the patella of symptomatic individuals such that the pain is decreased by 50% results in an earlier activation of the vastus medialis oblique (VMO) relative to the vastus lateralis (VL) on ascending and descending stairs. The VMO during stair descent activated 8.3° earlier than the VL, in the taped condition, as taping the patella not only resulted in an earlier activation of VMO but a significantly delayed activation of the VL (Gilleard et al 1998). This result has recently been confirmed by Cowan et al (2002), where it was found that tape leads to a change in the onset timing of VMO relative to VL compared with placebo tape and no tape.

Patellar taping has also been associated with increases in loading response knee flexion, as well as increases in quadriceps muscle torque (Conway et al 1992, Powers et al 1997, Handfield & Kramer 2000). When the quadriceps torque of symptomatic army personnel was evaluated in taped, braced and control conditions, it was found that the taped group generated both higher concentric and eccentric torque than both the control and braced groups. There was, however, no correlation between the increase in muscle torque and the amount of pain reduction (Conway et al 1992).

It has been suggested that patellar tape could influence the magnitude of VMO and VL activation but the results of a limited number of studies have not supported this contention (Cerny 1995).

PATELLAR TAPING

Patellar taping is unique to each patient, as the components corrected, the order of correction and the tension of the tape are tailored for each individual based on the assessment of the patellar position. The worst component is always corrected first and the effect of each piece of tape on the patient's symptoms should be evaluated by reassessing the painful activity. It may be necessary to correct more than one component. After each piece of tape is applied, the symptom-producing activity should be reassessed. If the tape does not change the patient's symptoms immediately or even worsens them, one of the following must be considered:

- the patient requires tape to unload the soft tissues
- the tape was poorly applied
- the assessment of patellar position was inadequate
- the patient has an intra-articular primary pathology which was inappropriate for taping.

If a posterior tilt problem has been ascertained on assessment, it must be corrected first, as taping over the inferior pole of the patella will aggravate the fat pad and exacerbate the patient's pain. The infrapatellar fat pad is one of the most pain-sensitive structures in the knee (Dye et al 1998). It appears that the fat pad, rather than the patellar tendon, may be the source of the primary pathology of many jumping athletes, particularly as there is a degenerative rather than an inflammatory process occurring in the tendon (Khan & Cook 2000). The patient's history helps differentiate patellar tendinitis (tendinosis) from typical fat pad irritation. The patient with patellar tendinosis must have a history of eccentric loading of the quadriceps muscle such as jumping or running downhill, whereas a patient with a fat pad irritation presents after a forceful extension manoeuvre such as forceful kicking in swimming or locking of the knees in power walking (see case study 1, below). Both patient groups have inferior patellar pain. With patellar tendinosis the pain is exacerbated by squatting and jumping. With acute fat pad irritation, the pain is exacerbated by extension manoeuvres such as straight-leg raises and prolonged standing (McConnell 1991). Therefore any treatment that involves quadriceps setting will exacerbate the symptoms.

CASE STUDY 1

A 14-year-old school student who was a fast bowler in the A-grade cricket team had been experiencing infrapatellar pain for the past 6 months. The pain was aggravated by bowling and was localized to the region underneath his patellar tendon, which would on occasions become puffy. He was no longer able to play cricket and the pain had recently started to bother him when he was climbing stairs at school. He was commenced on a regime of 250 straight-leg raises per day. Diligently, the boy commenced the treatment, only to find it was exacerbating his symptoms. On examination, the pain was reproduced as the knee of the symptomatic weight-bearing leg was extending, going up the stairs. Passively, the symptoms were reproduced by an extension overpressure of the tibiofemoral joint. The compromised structure was the fat pad which was being irritated by the inferior pole of the patella being pulled posteriorly during end-range extension manoeuvres of the knee (McConnell 1991, Dye et al 1998). The posterior tilt component was corrected with a lateral tilt, then a glide, by placing the non-stretch tape on the superior aspect of the patella, first in the middle of the patella to correct lateral tilt, and then on the lateral border to correct the lateral glide (Fig. 3.1).

The fat pad was unloaded with two pieces of tape, with each piece commencing at the tibial tubercle and going wide to both the medial and lateral joint lines respectively. The soft tissue was lifted towards the patella to shorten the fat pad (Fig. 3.2).

The patient was given specific training in weight-bearing for the posterior fibres of gluteus medius and the VMO using dual-channel electromyogram (EMG) biofeedback. As the patient's symptoms were dramatically reduced after the initial treatment, he was able to return to cricket. However, the tape failed when he was bowling, so the fat pad was no longer unloaded and the symptoms returned.

Figure 3.1 Tape from the middle superior part of the patella to tip the inferior pole out of the fat pad. Hypoallergenic tape is usually applied beneath the rigid strapping tape.

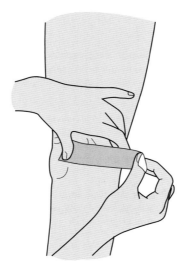

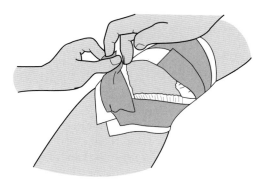

Figure 3.2 Unload the fat pad. Tape needs to commence at tibial tuberosity, coming wide out to the medial and lateral joint lines. The soft tissue needs to be lifted towards the patella. The therapist is aiming for an 'orange-peel' effect with the skin.

Video analysis of his bowling action revealed that at delivery his right knee locked into extension, causing a posterior displacement of the inferior pole of the patella, which impinged the fat pad with each delivery. With modification to his bowling action, so that he landed with a slightly flexed knee, his symptoms abated completely. The new bowling technique meant that the student could bowl even faster.

SPECIFIC VMO TRAINING

The current debate when rehabilitating the PF joint is over the type of strengthening of the quadriceps muscle. Powers (1998) concludes that, because there is no difference in the activation pattern of the VMO and VL in symptomatic individuals and the ratio of the two muscles is the same, generalized quadriceps strengthening is all that is required when rehabilitating patients with PF pain. However, this seems at odds with research on the effect of EMG biofeedback training and electrical stimulation of the VMO, which has demonstrated radiographically a medialization of the patella on the femur (Ingersoll & Knight 1991, Koh et al 1992, Cowan et al 2001).

It could be argued that individuals with poor mechanics need the VMO to fire earlier than the VL to overcome the abnormal tracking forces. Thus, the ability to fire the VMO selectively is a learned skill, which is enhanced by training. It has been found that 6 weeks of one session per week of physical therapy treatment changes the onset timing of VMO relative to VL during stair stepping and postural perturbation tasks. At baseline in both the placebo and treatment groups, the VMO came on significantly later than the VL. Following treatment, there was no change in muscle onset timing of the placebo group, but, in the physiotherapy group, the onset of VMO and VL occurred simultaneously during concentric activity and the VMO actually preceded VL during eccentric activity (Cowan et al 2002). Additionally, the VL can be inhibited by applying firm tape from mid-thigh across the lateral aspect of the thigh (Fig. 3.3).

In a recent study, Tobin & Robinson (2000) found that VL-inhibitory tape applied to aysmptomatic individuals decreased the activity of the VL relative to VMO during stair descent.

Figure 3.3   Inhibit the vastus lateralis by firmly taping laterally two or three times along the thigh.

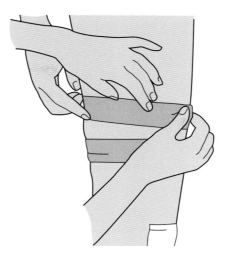

UNLOADING NEURAL TISSUE – A STRATEGY FOR MANAGING CHRONIC LOW-BACK AND LEG PAIN

Tape may be used to unload inflamed neural tissue. The unloading tape enables the patient to be treated without an increase in symptoms, so that, in the long term, treatment is more efficacious. The mechanism of the effect is yet to be investigated, but tape could:

- inhibit an overactive hamstring muscle, which is a protective response to mechanical provocation of neural tissue
- have some effect on changing the orientation of the fascia
- have just a proprioceptive effect, working on the pain gate mechanism (Jerosch et al 1996, Verhagen et al 2000).

The tape is applied along the affected dermatome region such that the soft tissue is lifted up towards the spine. The buttock is always unloaded (Fig. 3.4), starting medial in the gluteal fold, taping proximal to the greater trochanter whilst lifting the soft tissue up towards the iliac crest. This is followed by a tape which is parallel to the natal cleft, ending at the posterior superior iliac spine (PSIS), and a third tape joining the first two tapes from lateral to medial. A diagonal strip is placed halfway down the thigh over the appropriate dermatome and the soft tissue is lifted towards the spine (for S1 dermatome, see Fig. 3.5).

The direction of the tape depends on symptom reduction. The symptoms above the tape should be reduced immediately; the distal symptoms, however, may be exacerbated. If the proximal symptoms are worsened, the tape direction should be changed immediately (if worse, reverse), which should have the effect of improving the symptoms. Distal symptoms will be improved when a diagonal strip is placed midway down on the lower leg over the symptomatic dermatome and the soft tissue is lifted proximally (Fig. 3.6). Once the tissues are unloaded the patient can be treated without an increase in symptoms.

Figure 3.4 Unloading the buttock to decrease leg symptoms. The tape must be sculptured into the gluteal fold.

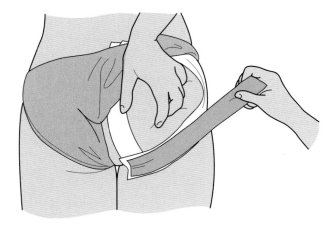

Figure 3.5 For S1 distribution of pain, the posterior thigh is taped, with the skin being lifted to the buttock. If the proximal symptoms worsen, the tape diagonal should be reversed.

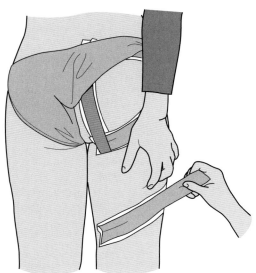

Figure 3.6 Unloading the calf to decrease S1 symptoms.

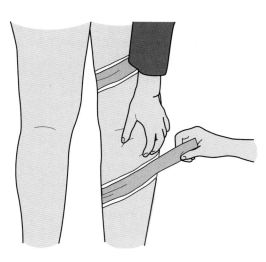

When managing low-back and leg pain, the clinician may need to change the treatment focus, so that the treatment is not just directed at the involved segment but addresses the contributory factors. Patients with chronic back and leg pain often have internally rotated femurs; this reduces the available hip extension and external rotation range, causing an increase in the rotation in the lumbar spine when the patient walks. The internal rotation in the hip also causes tightness in the iliotibial band and diminished activity in the gluteus medius posterior fibres, so the pelvis exhibits dynamic instability. The lack of control around the pelvis further increases the movement of an already mobile lumbar spine segment. It has been established that excessive movement, particularly in rotation, is a contributory factor to disc injury and the torsional forces may irrevocably damage fibres of the annulus fibrosis (Farfan et al 1970, Kelsey et al 1984). Therefore, an excessive amount of movement about the lumbar spine because of limited hip movement and control, in combination with poor abdominal support, may be a significant factor in the development of low-back pain.

Treatment of chronic low-back pain should be directed at:

- increasing hip and thoracic spine mobility to ensure a more even distribution of the motion through the body for functional activities
- improving the stability, rather than mobility, of the relevant lumbar segments. This involves muscle control of the multifidus, transversus abdominis (TA) and the posterior fibres of the gluteus medius. As it can take a considerable period of time for specific muscle training to be effective, tape can be used to help stabilize the vulnerable lumbar segments while the muscles are being trained (Fig. 3.7).

Figure 3.7 Stabilizing an unstable lumbar segment.

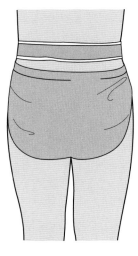

SHOULDER TAPING – REPOSITIONING OR UNLOADING

The shoulder, like the PF joint, is a soft-tissue joint whereby its position is controlled by the soft tissues around it. Poor muscle function, particularly around the scapula, and stiffness in the thoracic spine will severely affect shoulder function, making it susceptible to instability and impingement problems. In fact, most shoulder pathology relates to these two factors in some way. Impingement causes mechanical irritation of the rotator cuff tendons, resulting in haemorrhage and swelling, usually as a result of:

- encroachment from above – either congenital abnormalities or osteophyte formation
- swelling of the rotator cuff tendons – usually an overuse tendinitis associated with poor biomechanics, such as a faulty throwing or swimming technique
- excessive translation of the humeral head. Chronic anterior instability results in increased translation of the humeral head in an anterosuperior direction narrowing the subacromial space. Laxity of the anterior shoulder develops over time due to repeated stressing of the static stabilizers at the extremes of motion, e.g. the cocking motion in pitchers.

It is possible to increase the space available for the soft-tissue structures by repositioning the humeral head (Fig. 3.8).

The aim of the tape is to lift the anterior aspect of the humeral head up and back so that there is increased space between the acromion and the elevating humerus. The tape is anchored over the inferior border of the scapula. Care must be taken not to pull too hard anteriorly, as the skin is sensitive in this region and will break down if not looked after properly. The tape can remain in situ for about a week, depending on symptom reduction. Improving thoracic spine mobility and muscle training of the scapular and glenohumeral stabilizers must be addressed in treatment to ensure long-term reduction

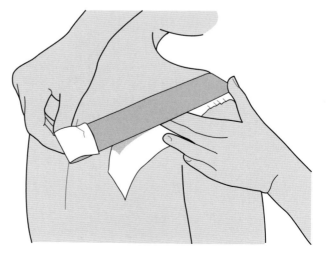

Figure 3.8 Tape to reposition the humeral head, decreasing the forward translation of the humeral head.

in symptoms. Athletic individuals with shoulder problems often have extremely poor trunk and pelvic stabilization, which also needs to be addressed in treatment to improve their athletic performance (see case study 2, below).

CASE STUDY 2

A 20-year-old elite female tennis player presented with right shoulder pain, which radiated slightly into the deltoid region. The pain was gradual in onset and had worsened as her frequency of training and playing had increased. She had been having symptoms for 12 months. She had had thermal capsular shrinkage surgery 6 months previously, and although initially there was some improvement in the pain, as soon as she tried to go back to tennis the symptoms returned. She was experiencing pain when brushing her hair, but she was still playing some tennis to keep her ranking. On examination, she had an arc of pain from 60° to 120° of abduction, pain on resisted external rotation testing and in the empty can position. On ligamentous testing, she had a positive containment test as well as increased laxity in the sulcus and posterior draw tests. She also exhibited laxity on ligamentous testing of the left shoulder. This patient was diagnosed as having multidirectional instability. Initially, the symptoms of instability and pain need to be minimized, by stabilizing the glenohumeral joint with tape (Fig. 3.9).

To begin with, muscle training should be directed at the posterior deltoid muscle to improve the centring of the humeral head in the glenoid fossa. As soon as the patient is able to control the humeral head position, rotator cuff muscle training can be incorporated in the rehabilitation programme, particularly working to simulate the service action, the symptomatic position and ultimately the core stabilizers so she benefits from the power generated from the legs.

Figure 3.9 Tape along deltoid in a fan shape to lift the humeral head up and stabilize the humeral head for atraumatic multidirectional instability. This tape should be applied with the patient sitting with the forearm resting on the plinth at 30° abduction.

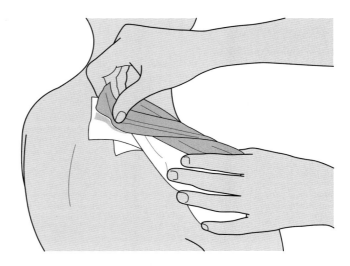

CONCLUSION

Musculoskeletal pain can be difficult to treat as the clinician not only has to identify the underlying causative factors to restore homeostasis to the system, but also has to ensure that the treatment does not unnecessarily exacerbate the symptoms. In some cases the clinician may need to unload the painful structures before commencing any other intervention. Tape can be used successfully to achieve this aim. Tape not only unloads painful tissue but it can facilitate underactive muscles as well as inhibit excessive muscle activity. The therapist receives immediate feedback from the patient as to whether the tape application has been successful or not. Tape can be adapted to suit the individual patient. It is readily adjusted and the tension can be varied. Tape is relatively cost-effective and time-efficient, so the therapist should be innovative and creative if symptom reduction has not been achieved, as tape can facilitate treatment outcome.

References

Bockrath K, Wooden C, Worrell T et al 1993 Effects of patella taping on patella position and perceived pain. Medicine Science in Sports and Exercise 25(9): 989–992

Cerny K 1995 Vastus medialis oblique/vastus lateralis muscle activity ratios for selected exercises in persons with and without patellofemoral pain syndrome. Physical Therapy 75(8): 672–683

Cholewicki J, Panjabi M M, Khachatryan A 1997 Stabilizing function of trunk flexor-extensor muscles around a neutral spine posture. Spine 22(19): 2207–2212

Conway A, Malone T, Conway P 1992 Patellar alignment/tracking alteration: effect on force output and perceived pain. Isokinetics and Exercise Science 2(1): 9–17

Cowan S, Bennell K, Crossley K et al 2001 Delayed electromyographic onset of vastus medialis obliquus relative to vastus lateralis in subjects with patellofemoral pain syndrome. Archives of Physical Medicine

Cowan S, Bennell K, Crossley K et al 2002 Physiotherapy treatment changes EMG onset timing of VMO relative to VL in subjects with patellofemoral pain syndrome: a randomised, double blind, placebo controlled trial (in press).

Cushnaghan J, McCarthy R, Dieppe P 1994 The effect of taping the patella on pain in the osteoarthritic patient. British Medical Journal 308: 753–755

Dye S 1996 The knee as a biologic transmission with an envelope of function: a theory. Clinical Orthopaedics 325: 10–18

Dye S, Vaupel G, Dye C 1998 Conscious neurosensory mapping of the internal structures of the human knee without intra-articular anaesthesia. American Journal of Sports Medicine 26(6): 1–5

Farfan H F, Cossette J W, Robertson G H et al 1970 The effects of torsion on lumbar intervertebral joints: the role of torsion in the production of disc degeneration. Journal of Bone and Joint Surgery 52A: 468–497

Gilleard W, McConnell J, Parsons D 1998 The effect of patellar taping on the onset of vastus medialis obliquus and vastus lateralis muscle activity in persons with patellofemoral pain. Physical Therapy 78(1): 25–32

Gresalmer R, McConnell J 1998 The patella: a team approach. Aspen Publishers, Gaithersburg, MD

Handfield T, Kramer J 2000 Effect of McConnell taping on perceived pain and knee extensor torques during isokinetic exercise performed by patients with patellofemoral pain syndrome. Physiotherapy Canada (winter): 39–44

Herbert R 1993 Preventing and treating stiff joints. In: Crosbie J, McConnell J (eds) Key issues in musculoskeletal physiotherapy. Butterworth-Heinemann, Oxford

Hooley C, McCrum N, Cohen R 1980 The visco-elastic deformation of the tendon. Journal of Biomechanics 13: 521

Ingersoll C, Knight K 1991 Patellar location changes following EMG biofeedback or progressive resistive exercises. Medicine and Science in Sports and Exercise 23(10): 1122–1127

Jerosch J, Thorwesten L, Bork H, Bischof M 1996 Is prophylactic bracing of the ankle cost effective? Orthopedics 19(5): 405–414

Kelsey J L, Githens P B, White A A 1984 An epidemiological study of lifting and twisting on the job and the risk for acute prolapsed lumbar intervertebral disc. Journal of Orthopaedic Research 2: 61–66

Khan K, Cook J 2000 Overuse tendon injuries: where does the pain come from? Sports Medicine and Arthroscopy Review 8: 17–31

Koh T, Grabiner M, DeSwart R 1992 In vivo tracking of the human patella. Journal of Biomechanics 25(6): 637–643

Larsen B, Andreasen E, Urfer A et al 1995 Patellar taping: a radiographic examination of the medial glide technique. American Journal of Sports Medicine 23: 465–471

McConnell J 1991 Fat pad irritation – a mistaken patellar tendonitis. Sport Health 9(4): 7–9

McConnell J 2000 A novel approach to pain relief pre-therapeutic exercise. Journal of Science Medicine and Sport 3(3): 325–334

Novacheck T F 1997 The biomechanics of running and sprinting. In: Guten G N (ed.) Running injuries. W B Saunders, Philadelphia, PA, pp. 4–19

Panjabi M 1992a The stabilising system of the spine. Part I. Function dysfunction adaptation and enhancement. Journal of Spinal Disorders 5(4): 383–389

Panjabi M 1992b The stabilising system of the spine. Part II. Neutral zone and instability hypothesis. Journal of Spinal Disorders 5(4): 390–397

Powers C 1998 Rehabilitation of patellofemoral joint disorders: a critical review. Journal of Orthopaedic Sports and Physical Therapy 28(5): 345–354

Powers C, Landel R, Sosnick T et al 1997 The effects of patellar taping on stride characteristics and joint motion in subjects with patellofemoral pain. Journal of Orthopaedic Sports and Physical Therapy 26(6): 286–291

Roberts J M 1989 The effect of taping on patellofemoral alignment – a radiological pilot study. In: Proceedings of the Sixth Biennial Conference of the Manipulative Therapists Association of Australia, pp. 146–151

Tobin S, Robinson G 2000 The effect of McConnell's vastus lateralis inhibition taping technique on vastus lateralis and vastus medialis activity. Physiotherapy 86(1): 174–183

Verhagen E A, van Mechelen W, de Vente W 2000 The effect of preventive measures on the incidence of ankle sprains. Clincal Journal of Sport Medicine, 10(4): 291–296

Chapter 4

Foot types, mechanics and therapy

S.R. Nickson and P. Madigan

CHAPTER CONTENTS

Types of first-aid padding 29
Common foot types 45

Appendix: Footwear 53
Further reading 57

This chapter aims to summarize the main mechanical problems encountered by the sports participant. Diagnostic clues are listed to facilitate decision-making by the practitioner. A range of quick treatments is given and methods of achieving them. Clinical padding and temporary insoles can be effectively combined with a range of tapings and strappings, described elsewhere in this book. Longer-term treatments are also discussed. Further reading is listed at the end of the chapter for those who wish to study the subject further.

TYPES OF FIRST-AID PADDING

Plantar metatarsal pads (PMPs)

Materials of construction

Uses

- redistribute load over a larger area
- alter the timing of load over a pressure point
- act as a locator for medication
- reduce friction over the metatarsal head area.

Adhesive

- chiropodist's felt (semicompressed felt), with or without adhesive
- open-cell, synthetic rubber cushioning (Swanfoam, Molefoam).

Insole and orthotic prescription

- Poron
- PPT

- Spenco
- Frelen insole base.

Method of construction (Fig. 4.1)

Outline of full thickness of pad in 5- or 7-mm semicompressed felt. The anterior border may extend over the second, third and fourth metatarsal heads or all five, depending on function.

Bevelling or skiving the borders of the pad will make it adhere better to the skin and prevent the patient feeling an abrupt ridge all round the pad (Fig. 4.2).

A more permanent pad can be attached to the underside of an insole base. The pad is cut to size, bevelled and adhered with double-sided tape. By adhering the pad to the underside of the insole, the need to cover the top surface is removed.

Mechanics of the pad and materials used

- Load is more evenly distributed over the surface of the pad, rather than being concentrated at the metatarsal heads.

- Load is reduced over a pressure point by making a V-shaped cut-out in the pad. This increases the length of time that surrounding areas are in contact with the ground (and reduces the time for the pressure point).

- Problems from skin friction, which occurs at the foot–shoe interface, are reduced by inducing friction to occur between the pad and the shoe.

Figure 4.1 Method of construction of plantar metatarsal pad.

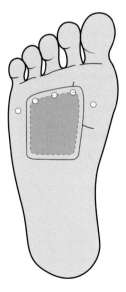

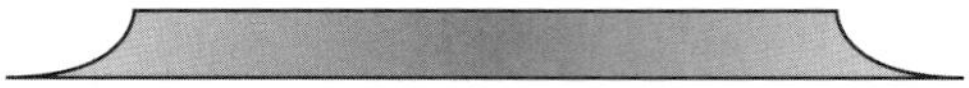

Figure 4.2 The borders of the pad are bevelled.

- If the aim of the pad is to alter loading, then chiropodist's felt should be used. Open-cell, synthetic rubber cushioning will assist in decelerating the forefoot and reducing force immediately before impact.

- They are easily cut to shape and can be adhered to the foot or to the insole of a running shoe. They are, however, short-term first-aid materials and, if successful, a similarly shaped insole should be constructed.

Variations on a theme: plantar cover pads

Uses

- cushion the whole metatarsophalangeal joint area (ball of the foot)
- redistribute load over a larger area
- reduce friction over the metatarsal head area
- alter the timing of loading over the area
- act as a locator for medication.

Materials of construction

Adhesive or replaceable padding

- chiropodist's felt
- open-cell, synthetic rubber (Swanfoam, Molefoam).

Insole or orthotic prescription

- Poron
- PPT
- Spenco
- Frelen insole base.

Method of construction

The pad may be adhered directly to a template made from thin cardboard or regenerated leather board (Texon) or thin EVA (Evalon) which is cut to the shape of the inside of the shoe. The patient wears this in the shoe for at least 1 week, to produce a dynamic imprint of the plantar surface of the foot. An alternative method involves inking the metatarsal heads and placing the foot and insole into the shoe. After the patient walks for a couple of minutes, the ink marks are transferred to the insole. From this, the metatarsal heads and centre heel can be identified and used as reference points for the pad. The pad is cut to shape, bevelled and adhered to the insole base and covered with a top cover or alternatively adhered to the underside of a Frelen insole.

Mechanics of the pad and materials used (comparison of the different materials required)

There is little to choose between the open-cell (Poron, PPT) and the closed-cell (Spenco) orthotic materials in terms of reducing pressure and force under the foot.

The open-cell construction of Poron and PPT is said to channel sweat and moisture away from the surface of the foot, thus keeping it cooler. The closed-cell neoprene rubber, Spenco, contains entrapped bubbles, or cells which are not interconnected, causing it to retain heat and moisture. This may be a consideration with middle- and long-distance events. Poron is available with an antibacterial additive to help combat a broad spectrum of the bacteria found in footwear.

Both types of materials are available with a preadhered nylon top cover which helps reduce friction.

Shaft pad

Uses

- to realign one metatarsal with the rest, e.g. in Morton's neuroma, apply to third or fourth metatarsal
- with a dorsiflexed first metatarsal and medial cuneiform, to bring the ground to the metatarsal
- to provide protection to a lesion such as a hard corn, overlying the metatarsophalangeal head (a crescent or cavity may be included)
- to provide protection to a lesion such as a hard corn, overlying the plantar surface of the interphalangeal joint of the hallux (big toe)
- to limit movement at the first metatarsophalangeal joint in a painful hallux rigidus.

Materials of construction

Adhesive

- chiropodist's felt.

Insole or orthotic prescription

- Poron
- PPT
- Spenco
- Frelen insole base.

Made in the same way as the PMP, and adhered:

- directly to the insole of the shoe
- to a Frelen insole base.

Mechanics

The shaft pad has a similar function to the PMP in that it provides protection to a lesion by increasing the available surface area through which pressure can be dissipated and by altering the timing during which the pressure is applied.

The surface area is, however, much smaller than that of the PMP, but it is a useful form of padding where space within the shoe is at a premium.

D pad or valgus filler pad

There are several variations of this pad.
Uses

- to reduce the effects of foot strain by filling the inner longitudinal arch or lateral longitudinal arch
- to facilitate the effect of an inversion or eversion strapping.

Variations

It may be constructed with a PMP to increase effective loading of the foot.

Materials of construction

Adhesive

- semicompressed felt.

Replaceable

- semicompressed felt on an elastic webbing or tubular elastic bandage.

Insole or orthotic construction

- Poron
- PPT
- Dense Plastazote.

Landmarks (Fig. 4.3)

- toes
- metatarsal heads
- base of fifth metatarsal
- level of tuberosity of navicular
- centre of heel.

There are several shapes described for this type of padding:

- The full thickness should extend from behind the first metatarsal head, following the curve of the long arch, and finish anterior to the weight-bearing surface or the heel. Some colleagues find that an extension on the medial side extending up to the navicular can be even more effective. Strapping the pad to the foot can incorporate any of the inversion strappings or plantar tension strappings described elsewhere in this book.

- The D shape is the other way round, with the straight edge extending from behind/posterior to the first metatarsophalangeal joint to the anterior aspect of the calcaneum and placed along the midline of the foot.

Figure 4.3 Landmarks of the sole of the foot.

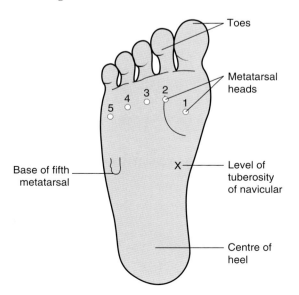

Figure 4.4   D pad.

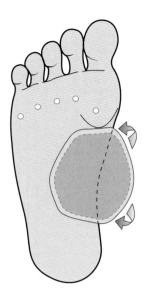

D pad (Fig. 4.4)

Mechanics

The available room for the foot to pronate is reduced by filling the arch of the foot or its corresponding space in the shoe. Pronation lengthens the foot and, if excessive, may strain structures on the plantar surface. Reducing the degree of pronation will give relative rest and support to the plantar structures. The pad may also be of benefit in compartment syndromes of the leg where muscles are working excessively to reduce pronation.

Heel pad (Fig. 4.5)

Uses

- sore heel – plantar surface or posterior surface (from heel tab)
- achilles tendinitis
- equinus and overuse syndromes
- location of medication
- soft-tissue trauma.

Materials

Adhesive

- semicompressed felt
- sponge rubber
- open-cell, synthetic rubber cushioning (Swanfoam, Molefoam).

Replaceable

- tubular bandage incorporating semicompressed felt or sponge rubber
- silicone rubbers as heel cups (Viscoheel) or incorporated into tubular bandage (Silipos, or self-made from a variety of products)
- sorbothane preformed heel pad.

Insole or orthotic construction

- Poron
- PPT

Figure 4.5   Heel pad.

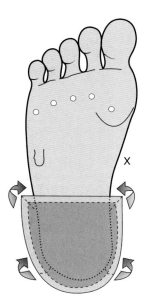

Figure 4.6   Method of
construction of heel pad.

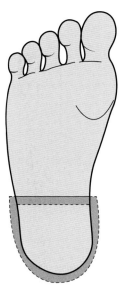

*Methods of construction
(Fig. 4.6)*

- Plastazote
- Sorbothane.

- Locate painful area.

- Cut full thickness of pad to follow margins of the plantar surface of the heel, extending to the anterior weight-bearing border. Do *not* forget to allow some extra material for a bevelled
  edge; this will make the pad easier to adhere to the foot.

- If necessary, create a cavity or aperture over the painful area.

- A combination of felt and sponge rubber can create a cushion effect directly over the painful area, whilst the felt will alter the timing of the loading.

This pad can be incorporated with ankle and arch strapping/taping and Achilles tendon strapping/taping.

Mechanics For Achilles tendinitis, heel bumps and equinus problems, the pad acts by lifting the heel and reducing the degree of dorsiflexion required at the ankle to achieve footflat. A fairly firm material is best and should be placed under the existing insole of the sports shoe.

For plantar heel problems, shock attenuation is improved and peak loading reduced with synthetic rubber (Poron, PPT) or viscoelastic (Sorbothane, Viscoheel) material.

Variations
- Medial/lateral wedge may be incorporated into a heel pad to alter the effects of excessive pronation/supination temporarily.

- Rose's bar – a rectangular piece of felt cut to conform to the anterior weight-bearing surface of the heel (Fig. 4.7) – has been used to alleviate the effect of plantar fasciitis and works well when incorporated into the specialist strappings for this condition.

Mechanics The felt bar supports the anterior part of the calcaneum and reduces strain on the plantar fascia during weight-bearing.

Figure 4.7   Rose's bar.

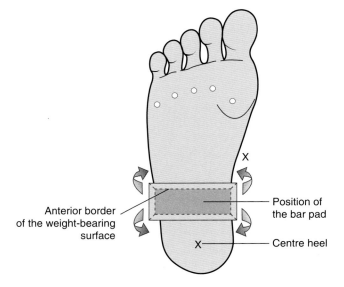

Anterior border of the weight-bearing surface

Position of the bar pad

Centre heel

Wedges   Uses

- Medial heel wedges (Fig. 4.8) are effective in foot strain and overuse syndromes associated with excessive pronatory forces.

Heel wedge

Lateral heel wedges (Fig. 4.9) are effective in cases of repetitive lateral ankle sprains and associated supinatory foot conditions. A lateral flare or flange may be required to overcome the supinatory forces.

Methods of construction

Adhesive

- Take a piece of felt that is just larger than half the plantar heel area.

- Bevel away the full thickness to accommodate the mid-heel weight-bearing surface.

- Adhere to inside of shoe or foot.

- Incorporate into an inversion or eversion strapping, depending on the result required.

Notes

Many sports shoes have removable insoles and wedges can be adhered to the undersurface of these with great effect.

Figure 4.8   Medial heel wedge.

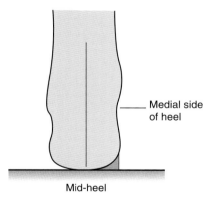

Medial side of heel

Mid-heel

Figure 4.9   Lateral heel wedge.

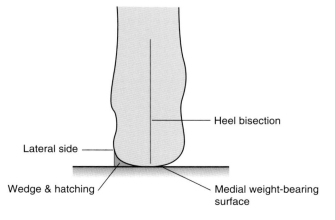

Heel bisection

Lateral side

Wedge & hatching

Medial weight-bearing surface

Insole or orthotic construction

If greater control is required than can be achieved by the aforementioned temporary measures, then an accurate non-weight-bearing foot cast should be taken. The preferred position is in the subtalar joint neutral position and is beyond the scope of this book.

Materials

Rigid and semirigid thermoplastics, incorporating wedges constructed from:

- closed-cell rubber
- Poron
- PPT
- EVA.

Mechanics

At heel strike the normal foot is in a supinated position. From this position it pronates to decelerate the leg and attenuate shock by unlocking the joints and allowing the bones to become loose and mobile. The foot must quickly halt this pronation and lock the joints, by returning to a supinated position, to become a stable weight-bearing and propulsive platform.

Problems occur when the joints of the foot, for whatever reason, are not in the right place at the right time.

See the section on common foot types, later in this chapter.

Dorsal pads

A range of protective pads can be used to great effect for single or multiple lesions.

Dorsal crescent pad (Fig. 4.10)

Uses

- protection for a corn, blister, laceration or pressure point
- vehicle for a medicament
- relief of shoe pressure

Figure 4.10 Dorsal crescent pad.

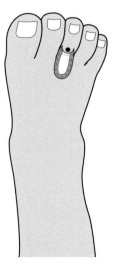

Materials Adhesive

- semicompressed felt
- sponge rubber.

Replaceable

- semicompressed felt. Sponge rubber
- tubular open-cell foam (polyethylene, e.g. Tubifoam)
- Silipos/silicone orthodigita.

Example • Hard corn, etc. on a lesser toe which is hammered or clawed. The full thickness should extend from just posterior to the lesion, down the long axis of the toe, finishing clear of the next articulation.

An underbevel (Fig. 4.11) protects the lesion and an overbevel blends the pad into the rest of the toe, improving adhesion to the toe.

The medial and lateral borders should match those of the toe. The bevelling extends into the interdigital spaces to improve adhesion, but does not interfere with toe function.

The pad may be held on by a T-shaped strapping or with tubular gauze if a dressing is incorporated into the pad.

Figure 4.11 Underbevel.

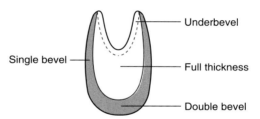

Variations Multiple dorsal crescents can be constructed to protect all or any of the lesser toes (Fig. 4.12).

Figure 4.12 Multiple dorsal crescents.

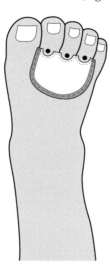

Notes

Avoid limiting extension of the toes and webbing by plantarflexing the toes before adhering pad and strapping.

Materials

Adhesive and replaceable

- semicompressed felt: 5 or 7 mm
- sponge rubber
- silicones.

Method of construction

Ensure a snug fit to each lesion. Measure the required width and depth of pad directly from the foot. Extend the main bulk of the pad proximally, so that the bevelled edge blends with the dorsum of the foot in the area of the metatarsophalangeal joints.

Strap the pad on using a 2.5-cm hypoallergenic tape halfway across the dorsal aspect of the second toe and taking around the plantar surface of the second toe and up on to the dorsum.

Notes

Do not allow the toes to be totally encircled, nor the tape to become too tight, as this may cause skin and circulatory problems.

Repeat for the fourth toe. Apply a curved base strap to the proximal edge of the pad, with the toes plantarflexed. This minimizes the drag effect of the dorsal skin.

Silicones

Various proprietary silicone putty compounds are available. The putty is mixed with a reagent and fashioned to the desired shape during its working time. The putty then becomes firm and will provide a useful and washable pad. For simple digital protection an elasticated fabric tube either containing a disc of, or fully lined with, a polymer gel (Silipos) is useful in cushioning prominent areas.

Digital props/splints (Fig. 4.13)

Uses

- single- or multiple-clawed, mallet or hammer toes which are flexible: their position needs modification.

Materials

Adhesive

- semicompressed felt.

Figure 4.13 Digital props or splints.

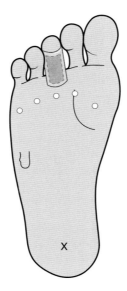

Replaceable

- semicompressed felt
- Poron
- PPT
- Plastazote
- Silicone.

Methods of construction: dorsal

The full thickness of the pad should extend from the distal interphalangeal joint proximally towards the toe web.

The bevel should protect any dorsal lesions. Medial and lateral bevels should extend to the sides of the second and fourth toes for secure adherence. The dorsal prop/splint can be combined with an adhesive plaster prop/splint to increase the effectiveness of both pads.

Mechanics

Digital padding is designed to protect lesions or other areas of pressure by increasing surface area, thereby reducing peak pressure. Some correction of digital alignment can be achieved where the problem is due to soft-tissue contracture, but this requires long-term management, which is best suited to bespoke silicone orthodigita.

Horseshoe pad (Fig. 4.14)

Uses

- to protect single lesions on very clawed or hammer toes, where minimal movement is available for correction.

Materials

Adhesive

- semicompressed felt

Replaceable

- semicompressed felt
- Poron

Figure 4.14 Horseshoe pad.

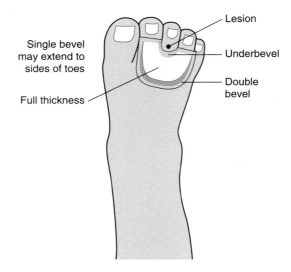

Lesion

Single bevel
may extend to
sides of toes

Underbevel

Double
bevel

Full thickness

Figure 4.15 Method of
construction of horseshoe pad.

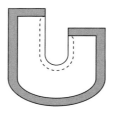

- PPT
- Plastazote
- Silicone.

*Method of manufacture
(Fig. 4.15)*

This pad is similar to a dorsal crescent but extended medially and
laterally to provide bulk and protection by using the adjacent toes.
The bevelling and extent of the pad are also similar.

It may be necessary to provide extra bulk immediately proximal
to the lesion. Toe straps can be used as for the dorsal crescent and a
base strap will be required to ensure good adhesion.

Replaceable pad

The above procedure is followed, incorporating an elastic net toe loop
for ease of use. Reverse the felt and cover the adhesive with tape.

Interdigital pads

Uses

- to prevent mediolateral compression
- to increase interdigital ventilation
- to realign toe relationships.

Materials

Adhesive

- semicompressed felt
- sponge rubber.

Figure 4.16   Dumbbell pad: view from (a) above; (b) below.

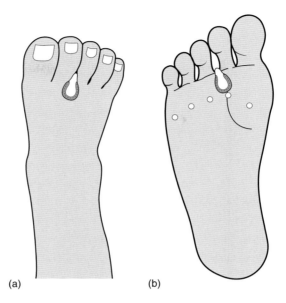

(a)   (b)

Replaceable

- tubular foam–open-cell
- silicone orthodigita
- Silipos.

Methods   The interdigital wedge is a trapezium-shaped pad, conforming to the dorsoplantar margins of adjacent toes. It extends from the webbing to the distal interphalangeal joint or further if the lesion is located distally.

It is bevelled all the way round and adhered to the toe with flexible strapping to prevent constriction of soft tissue and blood flow.

Mechanics   There is little space available between adjacent toes, particularly those which already show lesions due to mediolateral compression. Care must be taken to make the pad big enough to do the job, but small enough to avoid causing problems between other toes or between the fifth toe and the shoe.

These can be constructed from clinical padding. However, they are available ready-made from polymer gel (Silipos) or can be manufactured from one of the range of silicone putties to give effective orthodigita.

Dumbbell pad (Fig. 4.16)

Uses

- to realign proximal phalanges as they rotate and compress soft tissue on and over the metatarsal head, when a soft corn has been produced.

Method   The full thickness should extend for the total length of the interspace and be as wide as the interspace. The dorsal and plantar flaps

Figure 4.17 Dorsal and plantar flaps of dumbbell pad.

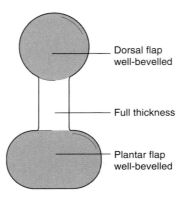

Dorsal flap
well-bevelled

Full thickness

Plantar flap
well-bevelled

Figure 4.18 Mechanics of dumbbell pad.

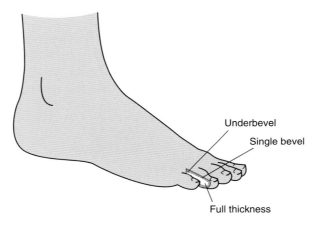

Underbevel

Single bevel

Full thickness

(dumbbells: Fig. 4.17) facilitate pad location and adherence. Tape may be used to increase pad security on both flaps.

Mechanics

The plantar flap raises the metatarsal and its proximal phalanx, while the dorsal flap, placed over the adjacent metatarsal, pushes it down, ensuring the realignment of the bony prominences which have caused the corn. The section of the pad within the interspace will act as an interdigital wedge (Fig. 4.18).

Apical pads (Fig. 4.19)

Uses

- protection of high-compression/friction areas.

Materials

Adhesive

- semicompressed felt
- open-cell, synthetic rubber (Swanfoam, Molefoam)
- sponge rubber.

Replaceable

- commercial apical toe covers in foam
- commercial silicone devices (e.g. Silipos)
- bespoke silicone orthodigita.

Figure 4.19   Apical pad.

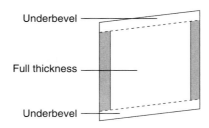

Underbevel ⎯⎯⎯⎯⎯⎯

Full thickness ⎯⎯⎯⎯⎯

Underbevel ⎯⎯⎯⎯⎯⎯

Methods   A strip of material is cut to equate to the distance from the dorsal distal interphalangeal joint to the plantar distal interphalangeal joint. The width is just wider than the toe to allow for bevelling.

Notes

Care must be taken to protect the nail plate and bed from the long-term effects of adhesive by either:

- stripping off the adhesive in this area or
- applying gauze, tape or appropriate material to eliminate the adhesive in this area.

Occasionally it is helpful to create a cavity in the pad directly over the lesion.

Apical crescent   This is a modification of a dorsal crescent pad and is most effective when made as an integral part of a plantar toe prop, otherwise the forces applying to the apex of the toe will still cause the toe to buckle.

Mechanics   The apex of the toe is not designed for weight-bearing and has little fatty padding. If the toe cannot be realigned, an apical pad of felt will increase the surface area over which load is distributed during ground contact and particularly propulsion. A degree of cushioning can be given to the apex with the use of cellular rubbers.

COMMON FOOT TYPES

Ideal foot relationships when subject is standing (Fig. 4.20)

Rearfoot varus (Fig. 4.21)

Definition   The neutral position of the subtalar joint is inverted to the long axis of the lower leg, causing the joint to compensate during weight-bearing by pronating to bring the medial side of the foot into ground contact.

Figure 4.20 Ideal foot relationship.

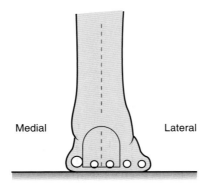

Figure 4.21 Rearfoot varus.

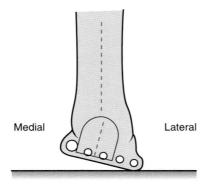

Clinical variations

Clues to look for:

Uncompensated rearfoot varus

- pinch callus on the border of the first and fifth metatarsophalangeal joints
- spin or rotational callus beneath the fifth metatarsal head
- lateral heel sprain
- soft corn or hard corn between fourth and fifth toes
- tailor's bunion (fifth metatarsophalangeal joint)
- callus under second and fourth metatarsal heads.

Quick treatment

- medial heel wedge to reduce the need for subtalar pronation as compensation
- PMP for forefoot lesions.

Longer-term treatment

- biomechanical assessment, gait analysis and orthotic-shoe prescription (refer to a podiatrist); modification to training programme.

Partially compensated rearfoot varus

This is where the foot can pronate but not sufficiently to allow full foot-loading in the time sequence.

Clues to look for:

- Haglund's deformity (heel bumps)
- inverted heel at mid-stance

- lateral heel callus
- history of lateral ankle sprains
- soft corn between the fourth and fifth toes
- tailor's bunion (fifth metatarsophalangeal joint)
- lesions beneath the first and fifth metatarsal heads (diffuse callus, not corns)
- hard corn on the dorsum of the fifth toe
- hip and low-back pain.

Quick treatment

- protective padding to dorsal and interdigital lesions
- PMP for forefoot lesions
- taping for lateral ankle instability.

Longer-term treatment

- biomechanical assessment, gait analysis, sporting style and modification of training
- footwear analysis, modification and advice (firm counters for rearfoot control)
- referral to a podiatrist.

Compensated rearfoot varus

This is where the foot has obtained full ground contact by pronating at the subtalar and midtarsal joints for longer than normal.

Clues to look for:

- mid-stance abductory twist of the foot
- Haglund's deformity (heel bumps)
- bulging talar head
- flattened medial longitudinal arch
- lateral heel callus
- lateral ankle sprain
- hard/soft corns on the fourth or fifth toes
- lesions or callus beneath all metatarsal heads
- hammer toes
- hard corn on the dorsum of the fifth toe
- hip and low-back pain.

Quick treatment

- protective padding to dorsal lesions
- combined PMP with valgus filler pad
- taping for lateral ankle instability
- footwear advice (firm counters for rearfoot control).

Longer-term treatment

- biomechanical assessment, gait analysis, evaluation of function in sport, orthotic prescription
- referral to a podiatrist.

Rearfoot valgus (Fig. 4.22)

Definition

This uncommon condition occurs where the heel is everted relative to the bisection of the lower limb when the subtalar joint is in its neutral position, causing internal rotation of the leg and pronation of the foot.

Figure 4.22 Rearfoot valgus.

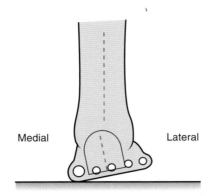

Medial   Lateral

Notes

The forefoot is also angulated in this position but, unless the patient walks in sand, the ground reaction forces cause maximal dorsiflexion of the first ray in particular.

Notes

It is unlikely that this foot type will allow patients to compete comfortably in their chosen sport!

Clues to look for:

- everted heel at mid-stance
- low medial longitudinal arch
- dorsal bump over the first metatarsophalangeal/cuneiform/navicular articulation
- lesion or hard corn beneath the first metatarsal head
- medial pinch callus at the heel and first metatarsophalangeal joint area.

Quick treatment

- if the foot is mobile, then use a combined PMP with a valgus filler pad and incorporate a wing shape around the plantar lesion
- inversion taping
- footwear advice and modification.

Longer-term treatment

- counselling on suitability to particular sporting activity
- biomechanical assessment, gait analysis
- orthotic prescription, where appropriate
- referral to a podiatrist.

Forefoot varus (Fig. 4.23)

Definition

This is where the forefoot is inverted relative to the rearfoot, with the subtalar joint in its neutral position causing the foot to function in a pronated position from footflat onwards. It is possible for the foot to compensate by abnormally pronating the subtalar joint.

Figure 4.23   Forefoot varus.

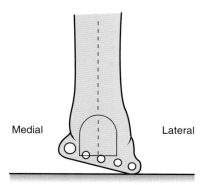

Medial   Lateral

Clues to look for:

Uncompensated forefoot varus
- propulsion off the lateral aspect of the foot
- mid-stance abductory twist of the foot
- mid-stance heel is *inverted*
- lateral heel callus
- spin callus beneath the fifth metatarsal head.

Partially compensated forefoot varus
- may propulse off the lateral aspect of the foot
- mid-stance heel is perpendicular or everted
- mid-stance abductory twist of the foot
- splayed forefoot
- hypermobile first ray (moving when it should not during gait)
- flattened medial longitudinal arch
- commonly, callus on medial heel border
- history of lateral ankle sprains
- tailor's bunion (fifth metatarsophalangeal joint)
- diffuse callus over metatarsal heads plus hard corns beneath the fifth metatarsal head
- hip and back pain
- hallux abducto valgus subluxations
- heel spur conditions
- lateral knee strain.

Fully compensated forefoot varus   As for both conditions described above, plus:

- bulging talar head
- intermetatarsal neuroma (Morton's toe)
- hammer toes
- pinch callus at the first metatarsophalangeal joint.

Quick treatment
- medial forefoot wedge
- symptomatic padding
- shoe advice (board lasted, firm counters).

Figure 4.24 Forefoot valgus.

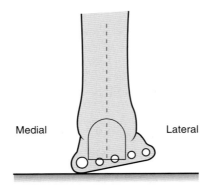

Longer-term treatment
- biomechanical assessment
- gait analysis
- orthotic prescription
- modification to sporting style and training programmes.

Notes

This is the most destructive foot type of all, because when the forefoot compensates by pronating to obtain ground contact, it has to bring the rearfoot also into a pronated position.

Forefoot valgus (Fig. 4.24)

Definition

This is where the forefoot is everted relative to the rearfoot, with the subtalar joint in its neutral position causing the medial side of the forefoot to come into contact with the ground very early in the gait cycle. The foot may compensate by dorsiflexing the first metatarsal to allow the lateral side of the forefoot into ground contact. If this movement is insufficient, the midtarsal and subtalar joints may supinate.

Clues to look for:

Rigid forefoot valgus
- Haglund's deformity (heel bumps)
- mid-stance heel is perpendicular or *inverted*
- spin callus beneath the fifth metatarsal head
- history of lateral ankle sprains
- soft corns between the second, third and fourth toes
- tailor's bunion (fifth metatarsophalangeal joint)
- tibial sesamoiditis
- medial knee strain
- hammer toes.

Flexible forefoot valgus
- mid-stance heel everted
- splayed forefoot

- hypermobile first ray
- flattened medial–longitudinal arch
- soft corn at the fourth and fifth toes
- tailor's bunion (fifth metatarsophalangeal joint)
- lesion beneath the second metatarsal head
- hard corn on the dorsum of the fifth toe
- hip and back pain
- diffuse callus beneath the second, third and fourth metatarsal heads
- hallux abducto valgus subluxation
- medial knee strain
- hammer toes.

Quick treatment

- lateral forefoot wedge to create full forefoot ground contact
- allow a crescent shape around the first metatarsal head to accommodate any corn
- stabilize heel with lateral heel wedge
- footwear advice and modification to provide good shock absorption.

Longer-term treatment

- biomechanical assessment
- gait analysis
- orthotic prescription where appropriate
- referral to a podiatrist.

Notes

This foot type is a challenge to the therapist as it can be quite difficult to achieve good results.

Equinus foot types

- talipes equinus
- metatarsus equinus.

Definitions

Talipes equinus   This is a fixed position of the foot or part of the foot, showing a plantarflexed relationship with the leg.

Metatarsus equinus   This is a fixed plantarflexion of the forefoot to the rearfoot at the midtarsal joint complex (Chopart's or Shaeffers' joint; Fig. 4.25).

The foot may attempt to compensate for equinus by pronating the subtalar and midtarsal joints and/or lifting the heel at an early point in the gait cycle.

Clues to look for:

Partially compensated equinus

- mid-stance abductory twist of the foot
- mid-stance heel *everted*
- splayed forefoot

Figure 4.25 Metatarsus equinus.

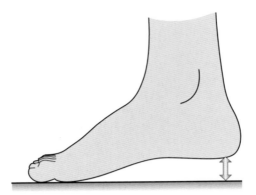

- spin callus beneath the fifth metatarsal head
- hard corn on the dorsum of the fifth toe
- lesions beneath the first, second and/or fifth metatarsal heads
- hip and low-back pain
- hallux abducto valgus subluxation
- lateral knee strain.

Compensated equinus   Same as above plus:
- bulging talar head
- hypermobile first ray
- flattened medial–longitudinal arch
- midtarsal joint break (seen on X-ray as midfoot bulge)
- early heel-off
- lesion or hard corn beneath the second metatarsal head
- lesions beneath metatarsal heads one to five
- hammer toes.

Quick treatment
- heel raise in shoe
- PMP with crescent to the second metatarsal head
- combined with a valgus filler pad if necessary
- crescent pad to the fifth toe
- footwear check.

Longer-term treatment
- biomechanical assessment
- gait analysis
- exercise programme for stretching, where appropriate
- orthotic prescription as necessary.

Leg–length discrepancy

Definition
- a small structural difference in leg length
- a functional leg length difference can be caused by the compensatory pronation for a varus or equinus foot type, or the persistent use of a banked indoor track.

Clues to look for:

- difference in malleolar/knee or hip position when standing
- excessive pronatory signs in the longer limb with supinatory signs in the shorter limb.

Measurement
- Measure the leg length for both limbs with the patient lying supine. The shoulders, hips, knees and ankles should be parallel to each other.

- Use the anterior superior iliac spine (ASIS) as a fixed bony point.

- Measure the leg length from the ASIS to the midpoint of the medial malleolus.

- Check each leg several times for accuracy.

- If there is a discernible difference, then this will be a true leg-length discrepancy.

Quick treatment
- Insert a piece of felt into the footwear, 5 mm for up to 0.5 cm leg-length difference, and 7 mm for up to 1 cm leg-length difference. If there is a larger difference in leg length, then serial heel raising may need to be tried over a period of weeks, while the patient adjusts to the changed position.

Longer-term treatment
- Footwear can be modified by incorporating a full-length lift to the outer sole, for a difference of up to 1 cm. This is the most effective treatment because the entire foot is short, not just the heel. Quality shoe repairers can do this without the shoes looking obviously different. Both sports footwear and everyday shoes can be modified by similar methods. It is worth enquiring from the supplier whether the manufacturer will do this, or if the shop can provide this expert service.

Mechanics
- A change in the leg length will affect the musculoskeletal system and the patient should expect some discomfort while the body modifies position and function.

APPENDIX: FOOTWEAR

Sports footwear

Despite the variety of shoes manufactured for specific sports, the basic structure of the shoe remains the same. However, varying construction methods offer differing degrees of control and support to the foot and this can provide a useful aid to taping.

In common with other footwear, sports shoes are made on a foot-shaped model called a last, of which there are three basic shapes: straight, semicurved and curved (Fig. 4A.1). The curve of the last is designed to reflect the slight inward curve of the foot.

The *straight lasted* shoe, which, despite its name, is slightly curved, will provide most support to the foot and is useful in the over-pronating foot where medial control is required.

Figure 4A.1   Left to right:
straight last; semicurved last;
curved last.

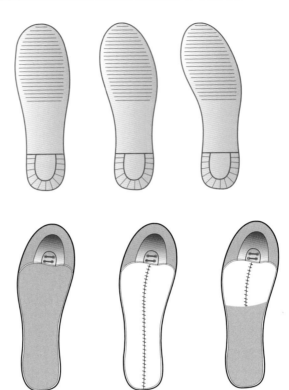

Figure 4A.2   Left to right:
board lasted shoe; slip lasted
shoe; combination lasted shoe.

The *semicurved lasted* shoe, which is the most common, offers a degree of medial support but without restricting foot mobility and is suitable for the majority of the population.

The *curved lasted* shoe offers the least amount of support to the foot and allows the greatest degree of mobility. This shoe type is useful in the rigid, high-arched foot which has limited pronation.

The various component parts of the shoe are brought together and glued or stitched around the last. The three most common methods used to manufacture the shoe exhibit differing characteristics in terms of foot support (Fig. 4A.2).

In the *board lasted* shoe the parts of the upper are brought together and attached to a board before the sole is glued in place. The use of a board, which can be seen if the insole is removed, gives a much firmer shoe with good stability and torsional rigidity but a consequent loss of flexibility.

The *slip lasted* shoe is constructed by stitching together all of the upper components to form a moccasin or slipper before the sole is glued in place. This gives a flexible, light-weight shoe which offers little control of the foot. Shoes made in this way have stitching from heel to toe which is seen if the insole is removed.

The *combination lasted* shoe is constructed by slip lasting the forefoot and attaching this to a rearfoot board during manufacture. The combination of the two construction methods produces a shoe which has good rearfoot stability. The rearfoot board and forefoot stitching can be seen if the insole is removed. The slip lasted forefoot is flexible and helps to reduce the weight of the shoe.

Square-box lacing

The square-box lacing method is designed to relieve the pressure caused by the lace as it crosses over from side to side across the dorsum of the foot (Fig. 4A.3).

Method

The lace is inserted into the two most distal eyelets on the same side of the shoe. Both ends are passed through eyelets on the opposite side before being fed upwards to the next two eyelets on the same side. The process is repeated until the final eyelets, when the ends are separated to opposite sides of the shoe.

Single-lace cross

The single-lace cross method is designed to pull on the toe box of the shoe and relieve pressure on the toes (Fig. 4A.4). It is particularly useful where pressure from the toe box has caused black toenails, blistering or lesions on the dorsal surface of the toes.

Method

One end of the lace passes directly from the most distal eyelet to the opposite most proximal eyelet. The other end of the lace passes upwards, from side to side, through each successive eyelet.

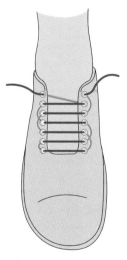

Figure 4A.3 Square-box lacing.

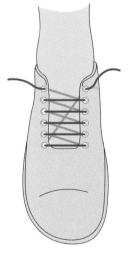

Figure 4A.4 Single-lace cross.

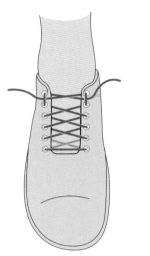

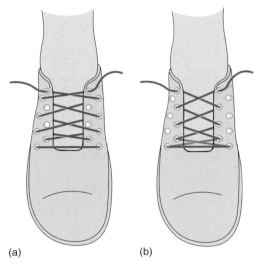

(a)   (b)

Figure 4A.5 Secure rearfoot lacing

Figure 4A.6 Variable-width lacing.

Secure rearfoot lacing

The secure rearfoot lacing method is designed to provide a more secure fit at the back of the shoe (Fig. 4A.5). This adaptation may be useful with a very mobile rearfoot or to improve security in a slip lasted shoe.

Method

The lace is inserted in the most appropriate method for the foot until the last eyelet is reached. The lace is then fed directly to the next eyelet to form a loop, before crossing to the opposite side, and is passed through the loop formed on that side.

Variable–width lacing

Variable-width lacing is designed to allow the lacing to be adjusted to accommodate either the wider or the narrower foot. Wider-placed eyelets allow the upper to be pulled more tightly for a narrow foot, while closer-placed eyelets allow the upper to accommodate a wider foot (Fig. 4A.6).

Method

Many shoes have a varied eyelet pattern to allow variable-width lacing. Where a shoe does not present a variable, additional eyelets can be added with the use of an eyelet punch.

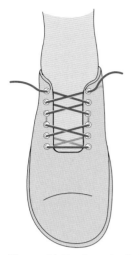

Figure 4A.7   Dorsal relief lacing.

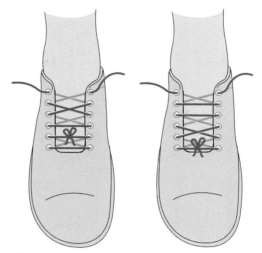

Figure 4A.8   Independent lacing.

Dorsal relief lacing

The dorsal relief lacing method is designed to reduce pressure over a particularly prominent area on the dorsum of the foot (Fig. 4A.7).

Method

The lace is inserted conventionally using the most distal eyelets and is passed upward, crossing from eyelet to eyelet until the lace reaches the prominent area. The lace is then fed directly to the next eyelet before continuing to be crossed until completion.

Independent lacing

The independent lacing method uses two separate laces and is designed to allow differing tensions to be applied across separate areas of the upper, ensuring an individual fit (Fig. 4A.8). It is particularly useful in the high-arched foot and where bony exostoses are present on the dorsum of the foot.

Method

While the shoe is being worn without a lace, assess which areas of the upper require to be at greater (or lesser) tension. Insert one lace from the eyelets immediately proximal to this area and work proximally. A second lace can be inserted into the eyelets distal to the first lace and worked distally. Alternatively, the lace can be inserted at the most distal eyelets and worked proximally until it reaches the first lace.

Further reading

Alexander I J 1997 The foot, examination and diagnosis, 2nd edn. Churchill Livingstone, New York

Anthony R 1991 The manufacture and use of the functional foot orthosis. Karger, Switzerland

Baxter D E 1995 The foot and ankle in sport. Mosby, St Louis, MO

Lorimer D, French G, O'Donnell M, Burrow J G 2002 Neale's disorders of the foot, 6th edn. Churchill Livingstone, Edinburgh

Root M, Orien W, Weed J 1971 Biomechanical examination of the foot, vol. I. Clinical Biomechanics, Los Angeles, CA

Root M, Orien W, Weed J 1977 Normal and abnormal functions of the foot, vol. I. Clinical Biomechanics, Los Angeles, CA

Part 2

PART CONTENTS

5. Foot 61

6. Ankle and leg 87

7. Knee 115

8. Lumbar spine 141

9. Thoracic spine 151

10. Shoulder girdle 161

11. Elbow, wrist and hand 183

12. Fingers and thumb 207

13. Stretch tape – many uses 225

14. Spicas and triangular bandages 229

Chapter 5

Foot

CHAPTER CONTENTS

Turf toe strap   62
Great toe taping   64
Hallux valgus   66
Foot support   68
Antipronation taping   70
Plantar fasciitis support   72
Plantar fasciitis taping   74

Medial arch support   76
Cuboid subluxation in dancers   78
Heel pain   80
Ligament and tendon support   82
Calcaneal motion control   84

Turf toe strap

J. O'Neill

INDICATION	First metatarsophalangeal (MTP) joint sprain.
FUNCTION	To stabilize and support the big toe in sprain of the MTP joint.
MATERIALS	Tape adherent, 2.5-cm porous athletic tape, 5-cm light elastic tape.
POSITION	The athlete should be sitting with the foot in a relaxed position over a table.

APPLICATION

1. Apply tape adherent.

2. With the foot and big toe in a neutral position, apply anchor strips to the big toe and midfoot (Fig. 5.1).

3. Apply four to six precut 2.5-cm strips (approximately 15–20 cm long) starting at the big toe and pulling down towards the midfoot anchor, covering completely the MTP joint (dorsal and plantar; Fig. 5.2).

4. Finish by covering the toe with two to three 2.5-cm strips. Cover the midfoot with 5-cm light elastic tape (Fig. 5.3).

CHECK FUNCTION

It is important to check function. The purpose of the tape is to stabilize the joint; if this is not accomplished, pain will result. Therefore the tape must be tightened.

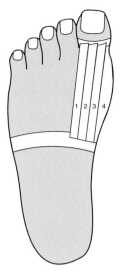

Figure 5.1

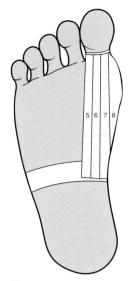

Figure 5.2

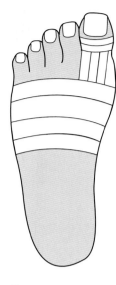

Figure 5.3

Tips

1. If pain is only in one movement of the toes (whether in flexion or extension), prevent only that movement. This allows for greater mobility of the toe.

2. Do not put the toe at an anatomical disadvantage – excessive flexion or extension – to prevent pain.

Great toe taping

K.E. Wright

INDICATION	Sprain to first MTP joint (turf toe).
FUNCTION	To limit excessive motion of the first MTP joint.
MATERIAL	2.5- or 3.8-cm adhesive tape, and 5-cm elastic tape.
POSITION	Ankle should be placed in neutral position and first MTP joint placed in neutral position.

APPLICATION

Steps

1. To begin the taping procedure, place the athlete's ankle and the first MTP joint in a neutral position and cover the nail with a plaster.

2. Apply two anchor strips:
   (a) Apply adhesive anchor strip around the distal aspect of the great toe.
   (b) Apply an elastic anchor strip around the midfoot (Fig. 5.4). This strip should begin on the dorsal aspect, go lateral, and continue across the plantar aspect to the midfoot medial portion, crossing the tape ends.

3. Four to six strips of adhesive tape should be applied to form a fan shape (Fig. 5.5). This will provide adequate support. Place fan-shaped tape from the anchor on the great toe, covering the affected area and ending on the elastic anchor at the midfoot (Fig. 5.6).

4. Using a continuous strip of elastic tape, apply a figure-of-eight around the great toe and midfoot (Fig. 5.7). This will aid in abduction of the first MTP joint and should assist in preventing excessive movement, flexion or extension of the MTP joint.

Figure 5.4

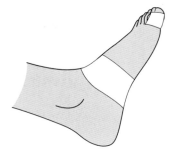

Figure 5.5

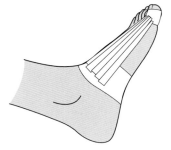

Figure 5.6

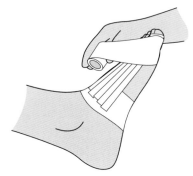

Figure 5.7

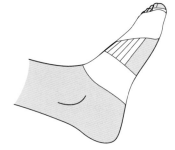

Hallux valgus

R. Macdonald

INDICATION	Pain in the first MTP joint due to valgus strain.
FUNCTION	To relieve the symptoms and allow walking in comfort. Helps to correct a mild deformity.
MATERIALS	Adhesive spray, 5-cm stretch tape and 2.5-cm rigid tape.
POSITION	Supine, with the foot over the edge of the plinth.

APPLICATION

Steps

1. Lightly spray the foot.
2. Using 5-cm stretch tape, attach to the medial side of the proximal phalanx of the great toe, distal to the joint line.
3. Anchor with a strip of 2.5-cm rigid tape around the phalanx to prevent slippage.
4. Draw tape back and around the heel, down the lateral side, under the arch, encircle the midfoot and finish under the arch (Figs 5.8 and 5.9).
5. Close off with a strip of rigid tape.

CHECK FUNCTION	Have the patient walk to check comfort.
CONTRAINDICATION	Ensure the tape is not too tight at the initial stage, as it may cause excessive abduction of the great toe.

Tips

Teach the patient how to apply the technique, as the patient can best judge the amount of abduction for comfort. The abduction may be increased little by little as necessary.

Figure 5.8

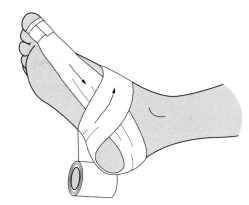

Figure 5.9

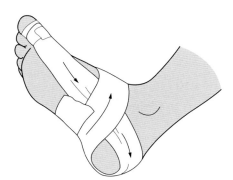

Foot support

G. Lapenskie

INDICATION

Foot pain, leg pain, retropatellar pain:

- plantar fasciitis
- tibialis posterior tenoperiostitis (shin splints)
- Patellar pain.

FUNCTION

To support the soft-tissue structures of the foot. To control the amount of longitudinal arch elongation (pronation) during weight-bearing.

MATERIALS

Adhesive spray, 2.5-cm tape.

POSITION

Put the athlete in long sitting. Position the foot with the subtalar joint in a neutral position and the first ray in slight plantarflexion and have the athlete maintain the position (during steps 1 and 2).

APPLICATION

1. Apply tape adherent on the dorsal and plantar aspects of the foot and behind the calcaneus prior to positioning the athlete.

2. Start the strip of tape on the lateral aspect of the foot of the fifth metatarsal. Bring it posteriorly around the calcaneus to the lateral aspect of the first metatarsal (Fig. 5.10a).

3. Repeat step 1, overlapping the tape by 2 cm (Fig. 5.10b).

4. Start a strip of tape on the plantar aspect of the first metatarsal head. Bring the tape posteriorly around the heel, crossing the arch to return to the first metatarsal (Fig. 5.11a).

5. Start similar strips of tape under the second and third metatarsal heads (Figs 5.11b and 5.11c).

6. Apply anchor strips. Start the tape on the lateral side of the foot; bring the tape across the plantar aspect of the foot. Push the thumb into the second, third and fourth metatarsal heads to splay the foot. While maintaining the splay, bring the anchor strip over the dorsum of the foot (Fig. 5.12).
   Repeat anchors, overlapping by one-half the tape width, to the tibialis anterior tendon (Fig. 5.13).

CHECK FUNCTION

Is the patient pronating during gait? Is patellofemoral pain relieved?

CONTRAINDICATIONS

Rigid foot? Pes planus?

Figure 5.10

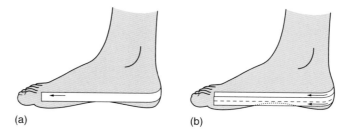

(a) (b)

Figure 5.11

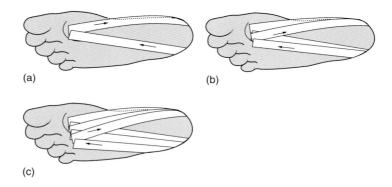

(a) (b)

(c)

Figure 5.12

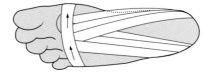

Figure 5.13

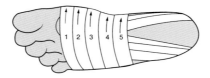

Tips

Heel pad is sometimes beneficial (Cyriax).

Antipronation taping

A. Hughes

INDICATION	Foot, ankle and lower-limb injuries caused by hyperpronation. A diagnostic tool to assess the value of functional orthotics.
FUNCTION	To limit the degree of calcaneal eversion which occurs early in the stance phase of the gait cycle. To assist plantarflexion of the first ray in late stance phase.
MATERIALS	3.8-cm rigid tape, 5-cm hypoallergenic tape, e.g. Fixomull or Hypafix, for application times that will exceed 4 h.
POSITION	Long sitting with the foot over the end of the bed. Foot/ankle complex maintained in neutral flexion/extension angle.

APPLICATION

Steps

Apply the hypoallergenic tape in the same sequence as the rigid tape to follow:

1. Apply two anchors to the forefoot, over, and just posterior to the MTP joints, overlapping by two-thirds (Fig. 5.14).

2. The initial support strip is taken with tension from the superomedial anchor back around the calcaneum, and down the lateral side of the calcaneum at an angle of 45° (Fig. 5.15).

3. The tape continues under the medial longitudinal arch to end on the superomedial aspect of the first ray. This will plantarflex the first ray when weight-bearing and reinforces the tape tension (Fig. 5.16).

4. Repeat with another support strip, overlapping the previous one by two-thirds (Fig. 5.17).

5. Finish with an anchor over the distal half of the first ray.

CHECK FUNCTION

When walking, the patient may feel a little unstable, as the ground contact surface area of the foot has been reduced with this taping procedure. The sensation quickly dissipates as the patient describes significant comfort, control and support with the technique.

CONTRAINDICATION Do not apply for plantar fasciitis in the absence of rear foot pronation, or rigid feet with a normal or high-arch/cavus foot.

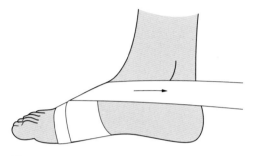

Figure 5.14

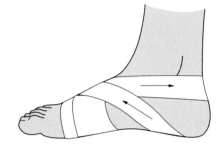

Figure 5.15

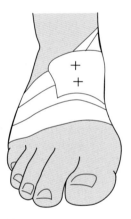

Figure 5.16

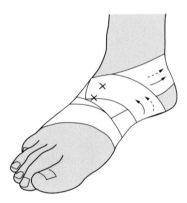

Figure 5.17

Tips

Apply this technique to the other side of the foot to promote calcaneal eversion, especially in the presence of a stiff subtalar joint.

Plantar fasciitis support

R. Macdonald

INDICATION	Longitudinal arch strain, overpronation (plantar fasciitis).
FUNCTION	To support arch and relieve strain on plantar fascia.
MATERIALS	5-cm stretch tape, 3.75-cm tape.
POSITION	Lying prone with foot in neutral position over the end of the couch.

APPLICATION

Support

1. Using 5-cm stretch tape, start on the medial side of the foot, proximal to the head of the first metatarsal. Draw tape along the medial border, around the heel and across the sole of the foot. Finish at starting point (Fig. 5.18).

2. Repeat the procedure. Start proximal to the head of the fifth metatarsal. Draw the tape along the lateral border of the foot, around the heel and back to the starting point (applying tension as the tape passes over the plantar fascia attachment to the calcaneus; Fig. 5.19).

Cover strips

3. Fill in the sole of the foot with strips of stretch tape. Start at the metatarsal heads on the lateral side. Draw the tape towards the medial side. Lift the arch up before attaching medially (Fig. 5.20).

Lock strips

4. Secure edges by applying a strip of 3.75-cm tape from the fifth metatarsal head around the heel. Finish at the first metatarsal head (Fig. 5.21).

5. Stand the patient up. Apply one lock strip over the dorsum of the foot to secure the tape ends (Fig. 5.22).

CHECK FUNCTION	Check that the great toe and little toe are not splayed. If they are, release edges.
CONTRAINDICATION	Rigid foot–pes planus.

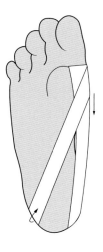

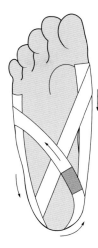

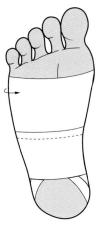

Figure 5.18

Figure 5.19

Figure 5.20

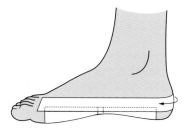

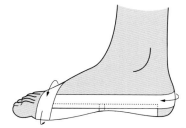

Figure 5.21

Figure 5.22

 Tips

Apply slight stretch to tape on application. A heel pad (Cyriax) is also beneficial.

For a sweaty foot, apply the last lock strips around the whole foot, making sure that the forefoot is splayed (weight-bearing) before closing the ends on the dorsum of the foot.

Plantar fasciitis taping

K.E. Wright

INDICATION	Plantar fasciitis.
FUNCTION	To aid in the reduction of stress on the plantar fascia and related foot structures.
MATERIALS	7.5-cm adhesive felt (moleskin), 5-cm elastic tape and 3.8-cm adhesive tape.
POSITION	Ankle in a slightly plantarflexed position.

APPLICATION

Steps

1. With the ankle slightly plantarflexed, apply the adhesive felt strip at the posterior aspect of the heel and firmly pull toward the metatarsal heads (Fig. 5.23). To eliminate binding, cut a V on both edges of the adhesive felt where the felt crosses the heel area (Fig. 5.24). Once adequate tension is applied, press the adhesive felt against the plantar aspect of the foot (Fig. 5.25).

2. Next, apply a 7.5-cm adhesive anchor strip from the medial aspect of the first metatarsal, around the heel, to the lateral aspect of the fifth metatarsal head (Fig. 5.26).

3. Apply 5-cm elastic tape around the midfoot area. This circular strip should begin on the dorsal aspect, go lateral and continue across the plantar aspect to the foot's medial portion, crossing the tape ends (Fig. 5.27).

4. Close off with a strip of tape.

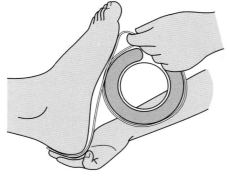

Figure 5.23

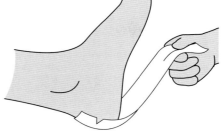

Figure 5.24

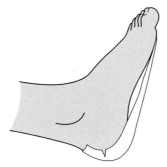

Figure 5.25

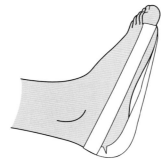

Figure 5.26

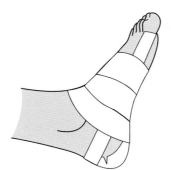

Figure 5.27

Medial arch support

R. Macdonald

INDICATION	Medial longitudinal arch pain or overpronation.
FUNCTION	To lift and support the medial arch and relieve stress on supporting ligaments.
MATERIALS	Felt or dense foam for arch pad, 7.5- or 10-cm stretch tape, 2.5-cm tape.
POSITION	Lying prone with the foot over the end of the couch.

APPLICATION

1. Measure the distance from the first metatarsal head to the anterior aspect of the calcaneus (Fig. 5.28). Cut an arch pad to fit this size and of appropriate thickness to raise the arch. Bevel the side of the pad which lies along the midline of the plantar surface of the foot. Sit the patient up on the couch.

Anchor

2. Using 7.5/10-cm stretch tape, depending on the size of the foot, cut a strip to wrap around the midfoot. Apply with minimal tension, with adhesive side facing out. Ensure closing seam is under the arch (this avoids seams under laces). Place the pad in position with the straight edge along the midline of the foot (Fig. 5.29).

Support strip

3. Cover with another strip of stretch tape, this time with the adhesive side innermost (Fig. 5.30).

Lock strip

4. Secure the seam with tape. Remove the entire support – turn inside out and close off the inside seam (Fig. 5.31).

CHECK FUNCTION	Allow the patient to move the support into position of maximum support.
CONTRAINDICATION	Not to be worn in conjunction with a shoe containing built-up medial arch support.

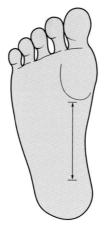

Figure 5.28

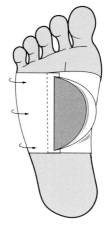

Figure 5.29

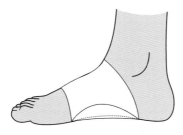

Figure 5.30

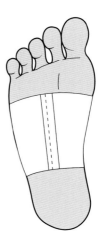

Figure 5.31

Tips

Removable support may be placed in the most comfortable position by the patient. Talcum powder will eliminate tackiness on uncovered adhesive mass.

Cuboid subluxation in dancers

R. Macdonald

INDICATION	Minor subluxation of cuboid associated with inversion ankle sprain in dancers, hypermobility of calcaneocuboid joint on plantar surface.
FUNCTION	To maintain cuboid in a stable position and stabilize the midfoot.
MATERIALS	5-cm, 7.5-cm stretch tape, 3.8-cm rigid tape, felt adhesive pad.
POSITION	Seated with foot over edge of couch.

APPLICATION

Steps

1. Stick the pad directly under the cuboid on the plantar surface of the foot with the outer edge bevelled.

2. Using 5-cm stretch tape, start on the medial side of the foot, draw tape back and around the heel.

3. Angle the tape down the lateral side, under the arch, pull up and encircle the foot to finish under the arch (Fig. 5.32).

4. Repeat the procedure starting on the lateral side of the foot, passing around the heel, under the arch from the medial side, and encircling the foot to finish under the arch (Fig. 5.33).

5. Hold in place with one or two strips of 7.5-cm stretch tape around the midfoot.

6. Tie down the edge with a strip of 3.8-cm rigid tape.

CHECK FUNCTION	Stand the patient up to see if the technique is comfortable.
CONTRAINDICATION	Refrain from activity for a few days to avoid a recurrent subluxation.

Figure 5.32

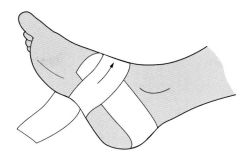

Figure 5.33

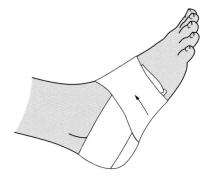

Heel pain

W.A. Hing and D.A. Reid

INDICATION   Heel pain, chronic plantar fasciitis, subtalar joint dysfunction. When a mobilization with movement (MWM) of the calcaneum has restored painfree function (this may be internal or external rotation, depending on which direction relieves the pain).

FUNCTION   Alters the position of calcaneum in relation to talus, thus correcting a positional fault.

MATERIALS   Spray adhesive or hypoallergenic undertape (Fixomull or Mefix). 38-mm strapping tape.

POSITION   Patient side-lying on plinth with the ankle relaxed in neutral position. If taping to maintain internal rotation of calcaneum, the patient lies with the affected ankle underneath, with the medial aspect of ankle superior.

APPLICATION   **Steps**
Calcaneum taped into internal rotation.

1.   The initial strip of tape is placed obliquely, around the back of the heel, while internal rotation of calcaneum is maintained (Fig. 5.34).

2.   Run tape obliquely and medially over the calcaneum.

3.   A second tape is placed over the first for effectiveness.

CHECK FUNCTION   When the patient initially stands, initial difficulty in walking may be experienced due to the repositioning of the calcaneum. Assess original painful movements (i.e. weight-bearing and gait). Movements should now have painfree full range of motion and function.

CONTRAINDICATION   If taping causes changes or an increase in pain. In particular with this taping, tape should be left on overnight, as it is often in the morning that the patient feels most pain.

Figure 5.34

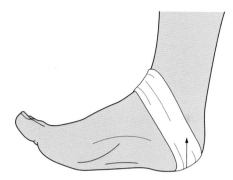

Tips

Easy to apply with the patient in the correct position; patients may be taught how to self-treat.

Ligament and tendon support

G. Lapenskie

INDICATION
: To be used to eliminate the posteromedial joint line pain following inversion sprain of the ankle:

  - Posterior tibiotalar ligament pain
  - Flexor hallucis longus tendon irritation.

FUNCTION
: To reduce the tension on the posteromedial aspect of the ankle joint. To reduce the strain in the flexor hallucis longus tendon during gait.

MATERIALS
: Tape adherent, 2.5-cm tape, 7.5-cm stretch tape.

POSITION
: Place the athlete in long sitting position with the foot suspended over the edge of the bed.

APPLICATION
: 1. Apply strips of tape from the plantar and distal aspect of the great toe to the mid-portion of the arch, ensuring that the plantar aspect of the MTP joint is completely covered. Anchor the tape by placing strips of tape around the distal and proximal phalanges of the toe, and across the arch of the foot. This prevents the toe from going into dorsiflexion (Fig. 5.35).

  2. Place the foot in a neutral position and externally rotate the foot (on a transverse plane around an imaginary longitudinal axis passing down through the dome of the talus). Place a piece of 7.5-cm stretch tape on the lateral aspect of the foot; pull the tape posteriorly around the heel to anchor itself on the leg (Fig. 5.36).

  3. Using the 7.5-cm stretch tape, anchor the tape around the foot and the lower leg (Fig. 5.37).

CHECK FUNCTION
: The patient should be able to run, toe-off, without pain.

Figure 5.35

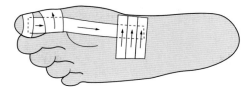

Figure 5.36

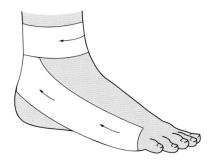

Figure 5.37

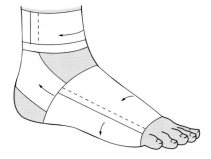

Calcaneal motion control

G. Lapenskie

INDICATION	Subtalar motion problems following inversion ankle sprain:

- sinus tarsi pain
- referred Achilles tendon pain
- reflex peroneal weakness.

FUNCTION

To maintain the subtalar joint in the neutral position by eliminating excessive calcaneal excursion.

MATERIALS

Tape adherent, 2.5-cm stretch tape.

POSITION

The athlete is placed in a supine position.

APPLICATION

1. Position the calcaneus in the desired position.
2. To avoid excessive varus motion, cut a piece of stretch tape 30 cm in length, and place the mid-portion of the tape on the medial aspect of the calcaneus. Bring the end of the tape close to the metatarsal heads under the arch of the foot, up the lateral aspect of the foot, over the dorsum of the foot, ending the tape by wrapping it around the lower leg. The piece nearest the calcaneus comes behind the calcaneus, anteriorly over the lateral malleolus, ending the tape by wrapping it around the lower leg (Figs 5.38 and 5.39).
3. Repeat step 2 (Fig. 5.40).

CHECK FUNCTION

Is the calcaneum stabilized when the patient is running (rear view)?

CONTRAINDICATIONS

None.

Figure 5.38

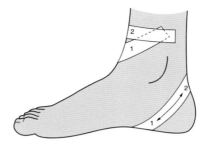

Figure 5.39

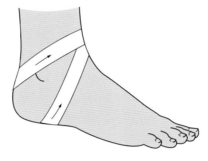

Figure 5.40

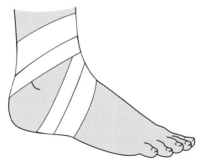

Tips

To avoid excessive valgus motion, start the tape on the lateral aspect of the calcaneus.

Chapter 6

Ankle and leg

CHAPTER CONTENTS

Acute ankle sprain – field wrap   88
Acute ankle sprain   90
Inferior tibiofibular joint   92
Achilles tendinopathy   94
Ankle dorsiflexion and rear foot
   motion control   96
Achilles tendon support – simple
   self-application   98

Achilles tendon support – two
   methods   100
Preventive taping for injuries to the
   lateral aspect of the ankle joint   104
Closed basketweave taping for the
   ankle   108
Heel locks for closed basketweave   110
Superior tibiofibular joint   112

Acute ankle sprain – field wrap

R. Macdonald

INDICATION	Immediate cohesive wrap for acute ankle sprain.
FUNCTION	To compress the injured soft tissue, help stop bleeding and contain swelling.
MATERIALS	7.5-cm cohesive elastic bandage.
POSITION	Seated with the leg supported, and foot in neutral position.

APPLICATION

For an inversion sprain.

Steps

1. Starting on the dorsum of the foot, encircle the foot once, by taking the wrap down the medial side, under the arch, up the lateral side. Before encircling the foot a second time, fold down a corner of the first turn so that it will be locked in place on the second turn (Fig. 6.1).

2. Continue the wrap from the dorsum around the back of the heel, over the dorsum again, down the medial side under the heel, as far back on the heel as possible (Fig. 6.2).

3. As you come up on the lateral side, rip the bandage down the centre to just under the tip of the lateral malleolus and wrap one tail around the front of the ankle and the other around the back (Fig. 6.3).

4. The cohesive bandage will stick to itself; there is no need for pins or clasps.

CHECK FUNCTION	If the patient is unable to weight-bear, a fracture must not be ruled out.
CONTRAINDICATION	Suspected fracture or total disruption.

Figure 6.1

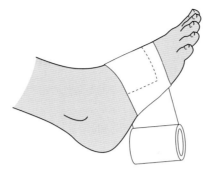

Figure 6.2

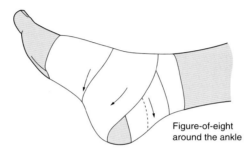

Figure-of-eight
around the ankle

Figure 6.3

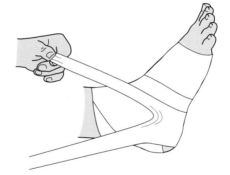

Tips

This wrap may be applied quickly and effectively on the field, as there is no need for scissors or clamps to close off the technique. It can also be applied over a shoe if removal of the shoe may cause further damage to the injured structures.

Acute ankle sprain

W.A. Hing and D.A. Reid

INDICATION	Acutely swollen ankle following inversion sprain.
FUNCTION	To provide a degree of support to enhance early weight-bearing and to reduce the swelling, apply compression and give some lateral support.
MATERIALS	38-mm tape, shaver, Mylanta, Fixomull, orthopaedic felt, compressive bandage (Coban).
POSITION	Patient sitting with ankle as close to neutral position as possible.

APPLICATION

Steps

1. Cut a felt horseshoe to fit around the lateral aspect of the ankle (Fig. 6.4).

2. Take a piece of 38-mm sports tape. Apply an anchor around the lower third of the leg (Fig. 6.5). This should not be tight or it will impede the flow of blood back up the leg.

3. Take another piece of sports tape. Attach to the anchor medially, working from medial to lateral to form a U-shaped stirrup. This keeps the tension toward the lateral side and prevents the ankle from turning in. In the acute stage, approximately two pieces of tape should be enough. Apply a final anchor over the top portion of the tape to hold the lateral tapes firm.

4. Finally, apply a Coban (cohesive bandage) over the taped ankle (Fig. 6.6). Start at the midfoot and apply a little more tension on the foot section, and reduce the tension as you work up the leg. This will ensure that the blood supply is enhanced in a distal to proximal direction.

CONTRAINDICATION Excessive swelling and patient unable to weight-bear following injury – assess for risk of potential fracture.

Figure 6.4

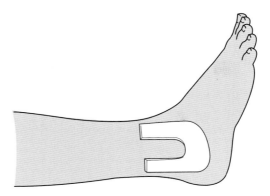

Figure 6.5

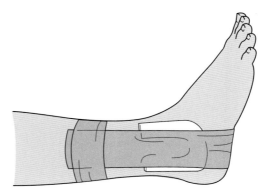

Figure 6.6

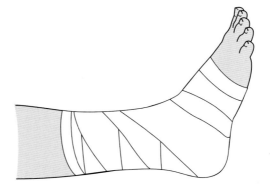

Tips

To enhance this, the use of a felt horseshoe increases the compression and supports the lateral ligament.
Also compresses the swelling around the lateral malleolus.

Inferior tibiofibular joint

W.A. Hing and D.A. Reid

INDICATION	Inversion trauma of the ankle resulting in positional fault of inferior tibiofibular joint. When a mobilization with movement (MWM) has restored painfree function.
FUNCTION	Corrects the positional fault of the fibula by repositioning it back on the tibia. The injury occurs due to the fibula being forced forward during excessive inversion action.
MATERIALS	Spray adhesive or hypoallergenic undertape (Fixomull or Mefix). 38-mm strapping tape.
POSITION	Ankle in neutral position. Patient lying supine on plinth.

APPLICATION

Steps

1. Aim of taping is to glide fibula dorsocranially.

2. Apply and maintain MWM to the distal fibula.

3. Tape starts anterolaterally over the distal end of the fibula and lies obliquely (Fig. 6.7).

4. Direct the tape in a posterosuperior direction, making sure to lay the tape over the Achilles, to end anteromedially on the tibia (Fig. 6.8).

CHECK FUNCTION	Taping should not restrict ankle movements. Assess original painful movements (ankle inversion, gait). Movements should now be painfree with full range of motion and function.
CONTRAINDICATION	In acute stages ensure that taping does not prevent a reduction in swelling by being too tight or encompassing the leg. Also rule out the possibility of an avulsion fracture of the fibula.

Figure 6.7

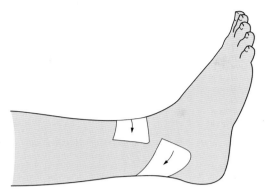

Figure 6.8

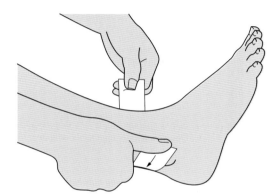

Tips

Never tape the foot in eversion, as this will inhibit normal ankle movement and thus slow down the healing process. If taping causes changes or an increase in pain, it should not be left on for >48 h, and should be removed at any hint of skin irritation.

Achilles tendinopathy

W.A. Hing and D.A. Reid

INDICATION	Pain on the medial or lateral aspect of the tendon. When a MWM has restored painfree function.
FUNCTION	Utilized when the patient has pronated or supinated feet. In the case of pronated feet (when viewed from behind), the Achilles tendon may appear convex medially and thus more vulnerable to strain. Taping reduces the loading on the medial aspect of the tendon by making the tendon concave medially, alters the way the foot weight-bears and changes the tracking of the tendon/muscle.
MATERIALS	Spray adhesive or hypoallergenic undertape (Fixomull or Mefix). 38-mm strapping tape, shaver.
POSITION	Patient lying prone with foot relaxed over edge of plinth.

APPLICATION

Steps

Taping for medial Achilles tendon pain:

1. Apply tape to the medial aspect of the tendon running posteriorly.

2. Place finger on the medial aspect of the tendon over the tape and apply lateral pressure to concave the tendon medially, thus correcting the convexity.

3. Direct the tape posteriorly, 'laying on' over the tendon and continuing around the lateral aspect of the ankle to finish anteriorly (Fig. 6.9).

4. Once the initial piece of tape has been applied, lay a second piece directly over the first.

CHECK FUNCTION

Tendon should appear in neutral, or concave to the side of the painful tendon once taped.

Assess original painful movements (i.e. walking, toe-raise). Movements should now have painfree full range of motion and function.

Figure 6.9

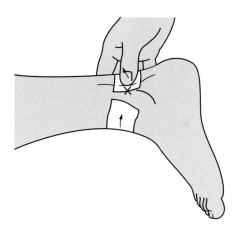

CONTRAINDICATION   If taping causes changes or an increase in pain, tape should not be left on for >48 h, and should be removed at any hint of skin irritation.

Tips

Use Mylanta (this is a stomach antacid which neutralizes the acidity of the tape: use extra strength) on the skin to avoid an adverse skin reaction to the tape. Before applying the tape, brush off the surface powder that appears when the Mylanta dries.

This procedure is easy to apply with the patient in the correct position, so a family member could be taught to do the taping. This would allow the tape to be removed at night and reapplied in the morning, preventing the risk of an adverse skin reaction.

Ankle dorsiflexion and rear foot motion control

G. Lapenskie

INDICATION

Achilles tendon problems, subtalar motion problems:

- Achilles tendinitis
- subtalar instabilities following inversion ankle sprains.

FUNCTION

To control the amount of dorsiflexion of the ankle. To maintain the position of the rear foot during weight-bearing.

MATERIALS

Adhesive spray, 3.8-cm tape, 7.5-cm stretch tape.

POSITION

Put the athlete prone, lying with the foot extending beyond the bed. Place the rear foot in the desired position.

APPLICATION

Steps

1. Start a piece of 3.8-cm tape on the distal third, medial aspect of the leg. Bring the tape down and laterally over the lateral aspect of the heel, under the arch, to the dorsum of the foot (Fig. 6.10).

2. Start a second piece of 3.8-cm tape on the lateral aspect of the leg at the distal third of the leg. Bring the tape medially over the medial aspect of the heel, under the arch, to the dorsum of the foot (Fig. 6.11).

3. Repeat the sequence three times in each direction, slightly overlapping towards the midline of the leg (Fig. 6.12).

Anchor strips

4. Anchor the proximal and distal ends of the tape with the 7.5-cm stretch tape (Fig. 6.13).

CHECK FUNCTION

Is the tape irritating the Achilles tendon during gait?

CONTRAINDICATIONS

Acute peritendinitis.

Tips

Heel cushion under heel.

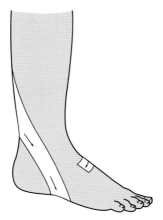

Figure 6.10

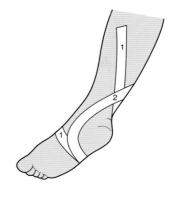

Figure 6.11

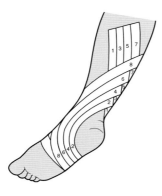

Figure 6.12

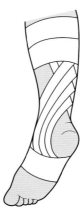

Figure 6.13

Achilles tendon support – simple self–application

R. Macdonald

INDICATION	Achilles tendon strain.
MATERIALS	Adhesive spray, gauze square, felt pad, 7.5-cm stretch tape, 3.8-cm tape.
POSITION	Sitting, knees bent with foot relaxed on couch.
APPLICATION	Spray and apply protection pad to Achilles tendon.
Support strip	Cut a 30-cm strip of 7.5-cm stretch tape and split the ends into four tails about 10 cm deep. Place the heel in the centre of the strip and wrap the front tails around the midfoot (Fig. 6.14). Wrap the other two tails around the lower leg above the Achilles tendon, pulling the foot into plantarflexion. Place the protective felt pad at the V-junction of the rear tape split.
Lock strips	Apply anchors to lock down the ends.
CHECK FUNCTION	Ensure the Achilles tendon is protected.

Figure 6.14

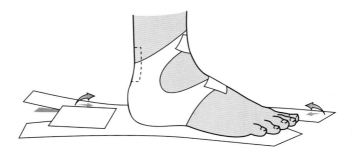

Tips

Place heel pads under the heels.

Achilles tendon support – two methods

O. Rouillon

INDICATIONS
1. simple method – using stretch tape, non-weight-bearing, preventive.
2. to stabilize the rear foot, preventive.
3. rigid tape method – for sport.

Prophylactically, it is better to use type 1 or 2.

METHOD 1 – SIMPLE METHOD

MATERIALS   Gauze squares, lubricant, adhesive spray, prowrap, scissors (blunt-ended), 8- and 6-cm stretch tape.

POSITION   Sitting with the leg over the end of the couch.

APPLICATION   Lubricated gauze square over the Achilles tendon. Adhesive spray on the leg. Prowrap from foot to top of calf.

1. Using 6-cm stretch, apply anchor around the foot, proximal to the metatarsal heads, and another around the proximal end of the calf.

SECOND POSITION   Prone lying

2. Using 6-cm stretch tape, attach it to the distal anchor on the plantar surface. Pass over the calcaneum and Achilles tendon and attach to the posterior aspect of proximal anchor, with tension (Fig. 6.15).

3. Attach two more strips to the plantar surface, bisecting strip 1. Pass upwards to the proximal anchor with the inner edge travelling along the centre of strip 1, one each on the medial and lateral aspects (Fig. 6.16).

4. Using 8-cm stretch tape, attach it centrally on the distal anchor. Proceed as before up the posterior aspect of the calf. Before attaching, cut two tails at the proximal end, 20 cm long. Separate at the musculotendinous junction of the triceps surae; attach to the proximal anchor medially and laterally to the previous strips (Fig. 6.17).

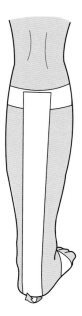

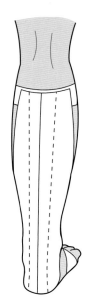

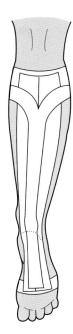

Figure 6.15   Figure 6.16   Figure 6.17

Finish by repeating the original anchors (lock strips) proximal and distal.

METHOD 2 – FOR REAR FOOT STABILIZATION

MATERIALS Two gauze squares for the Achilles tendon and the anterior foot tendons, spray, prowrap and lubricant.

POSITION Proceed as for method 1.

APPLICATION Using 6-cm stretch tape, apply two anchors, one around the midfoot, the second around the proximal calf.

Anchors

1. Cut three strips of 6-cm tape, measuring from the proximal to the distal anchor. Attach to the proximal anchor. Cut two tails on the distal end, 10 cm long. Split the tails to just above the Achilles tendon.

2. Apply the medial tail over the medial malleoli under the calcaneum, up the lateral side of the foot to finish on the dorsum. Repeat with the other tail, passing over the lateral aspect.

3. Apply the second and third strips in the same manner, superimposed on strip 1, moving anteriorly (Fig. 6.18).

Finish Apply 6-cm cohesive wrap.

Tips

Cut three strips before you start.

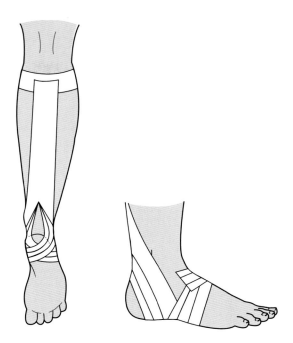

Figure 6.18

Preventive taping for injuries to the lateral aspect of the ankle joint

D. Reese

INDICATIONS

- prevention of injuries caused by foot inversion
- strain to the peroneus tendons
- slight or healing sprain to the anterior talofibular ligament and/or calcaneofibular ligament.

FUNCTION

To give support to the lateral aspect of the ankle by a combination of mechanical support supplied by the tape and its interface with the anchors and proprioceptive response triggered by the pull of the skin when supinating the foot during activity.

MATERIALS

3.75/5-cm tape, depending on the size of the ankle. Underwrap and one or two gauze squares with lubricant.

POSITION

Patient sitting with the foot over the end of the bench or the lower leg supported by a taping support under the lower leg.

APPLICATION

The patient should be clean, dry and shaved in the area to be taped. Start by having the patient actively holding the foot neutrally at the anatomical 0 position for the foot (or 90°). For patients who sweat profusely or who will be active in a wet environment, it is recommended to use adhesive spray. Apply the underwrap in a figure-of-eight around the ankle joint, covering the lower aspect of the Achilles tendon and the dorsal aspect of the joint, or place two heel-and-lace pads or gauze squares with lubricant (one placed on the Achilles tendon, the other at the dorsal junction between the malleoli and the talus).

Anchors

Anchors 1, 2 and 3 should be placed starting approximately 5 cm distal to the belly of the gastrocnemius. Apply the tape so that it conforms to the natural angle of the lower leg. Overlap distally approximately one-quarter of the width of the first anchor. The bottom part of the last anchor should lie just proximal to the malleoli. Check to see that the anchors do not constrict the range of motion (Fig. 6.19).

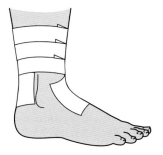

Figure 6.19

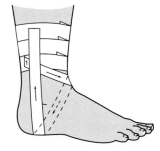

Figure 6.20

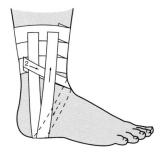

Figure 6.21

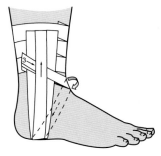

Figure 6.22

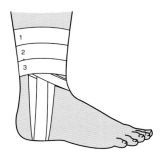

Figure 6.23

Support

1. The first support should start just proximal to the lateral malleolus. It should be angled downwards towards the posterior aspect of the calcaneus and then pulled tautly upwards, covering the back half of the lateral malleolus and continuing upwards to the level of the first anchor (Fig. 6.20).

2. The second support starts proximal to the first support. The angle downwards should be directed so that, as it passes anteriorly to the medial malleolus, it should lie directly on top of the first support, continuing on the calcaneus, to be pulled tautly upwards covering the anterior half of the malleolus, and creating a V-formation together with the first support (Fig. 6.21).

3. The third support is placed in the centre of the first two. Pull tautly upwards, covering the malleolus (Fig. 6.22).

Anchor lock

Apply three more anchors over the originals (Fig. 6.23).

Arch support

The arch support should start proximal to the medial malleolus. It passes downwards over the lateral aspect of the foot and then is pulled tautly upwards, finishing at the apex of the medial arch (Fig. 6.24).

Heal lock

The lateral heel lock starts proximal to the *lateral malleolus*. It should be angled downwards towards the posterior aspect of calcaneum and then pulled tautly upwards, covering calcaneum laterally. It continues over the medial malleolus, angled upwards, and finishes parallel to the start (Fig 6.25).

CHECK FUNCTION

Once the supports have been applied, hold them manually in place and ask the patient if he or she is receiving the desired support. If not, adjust the supports before applying the anchor locks.

CONTRAINDICATIONS

Application should be avoided when the patient has a swollen joint.

Tips

Best applied directly to the skin. When applying the supports be careful to keep proximal to the base of the fifth metatarsal.

Figure 6.24

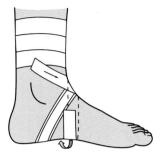

Figure 6.25

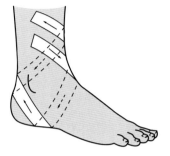

Closed basketweave taping for the ankle

R. Macdonald

INDICATION	Ankle inversion sprain.
FUNCTION	To support lateral ligaments without limiting motion unnecessarily.
MATERIALS	Gauze squares or heel-and-lace pads, petroleum jelly, adhesive spray, underwrap, 3.75-cm tape.
POSITION	Patient sitting on couch/bench with foot and ankle over edge. Foot in dorsiflexion and everted.
APPLICATION	Spray area. Apply lubricated gauze squares over pressure areas (extensor tendons and Achilles tendon). Apply a single layer of underwrap (Fig. 6.26).
Anchors	Apply anchors to the leg about 10 cm above the malleoli, conforming to the shape of the leg and to the midfoot. These anchors should overlap underwrap by 2 cm and adhere directly to the skin (Fig. 6.27).
Support	Apply first the vertical stirrup, starting on the medial side of the anchor. Continue down posterior to the medial malleolus, under the heel and up the lateral side (with tension). Attach to the anchor. (Do not mould to leg.)
Horizontal strips	Apply a horizontal (Gibney) strip. Start on the lateral side of the anchor, continue around the heel and attach to the medial side of the foot anchor (Fig. 6.28). Continue to apply vertical and horizontal strips alternately until the ankle is covered. Ensure each strip overlaps the preceding one by one-third (Fig. 6.29).
Lock strips	Fill in with locking strips between anchors (Fig. 6.30).
CHECK FUNCTION	Is it supportive, but not too tight?

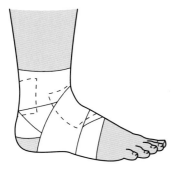

Figure 6.26

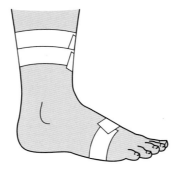

Figure 6.27

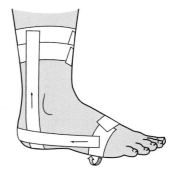

Figure 6.28

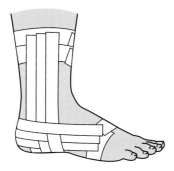

Figure 6.29

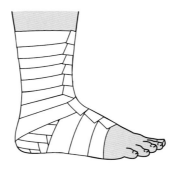

Figure 6.30

CONTRAINDICATIONS   Swelling, inflammation, bleeding.

Tips

Mould with hands to warm and set.

Heel locks for closed basketweave

R. Macdonald

INDICATION   Ankle sprain.

FUNCTION   To provide extra support with double heel lock.

MATERIALS   3.8-cm tape.

APPLICATION
1. Start on the medial side of the leg. Angle tape down over the lateral side, behind and under the heel, pulling up and out (Fig. 6.31).

2. Continue over the dorsum of the foot, back over the medial malleolus behind the heel (Fig. 6.32).

3. Continue down under the heel, pulling up to the medial side (Fig. 6.33).

4. Proceed across the front of the foot and finish high on the lateral side (Fig. 6.34).

Tips

For the novice, two single heel locks are easier to apply. The first starts on the medial side, and the second on the lateral side.

Figure 6.31

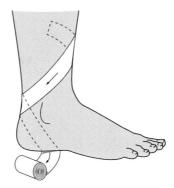

Figure 6.32

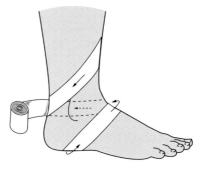

Figure 6.33

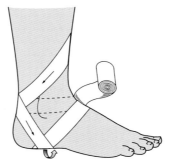

Figure 6.34

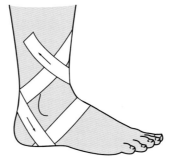

Superior tibiofibular joint

W.A. Hing and D.A. Reid

INDICATION	Posterolateral knee pain, commonly with weight-bearing and gait, especially walking down stairs or slopes. Patients with remnants of leg pain down the lateral border of the lower leg to the foot. Note the previously described conditions in which MWMs are painfree and successful.
FUNCTION	Repositions the fibula head forward on the tibia. Also, possibly altering tension on nerve responsible for pain, (e.g. common peroneal nerve).
MATERIALS	Spray adhesive or hypoallergenic undertape (Fixomull or Mefix). 38-mm strapping tape, shaver.
POSITION	Patient standing with affected knee flexed and foot placed on a chair.

APPLICATION

Steps

1. Place tape over superior head of the fibula.

2. Apply and maintain a MWM to superior fibula head (Fig. 6.35).

3. In an anterior direction, wrap tape obliquely across the front of the tibia.

4. Tape will end on the medial side of the tibia (Fig. 6.36).

CHECK FUNCTION	Ensure there is full range of motion at the knee, and that the tape is not constricting the gastrocnemius muscles. Assess original painful movements (knee flexion, stepping down off a step). Movements should now have painfree full range of motion and function.
CONTRAINDICATION	If taping causes changes or an increase in pain. Also tape should not be left on for >48 h, and should be removed at any hint of skin irritation.

Figure 6.35

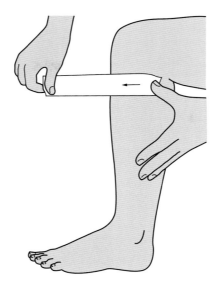

Figure 6.36

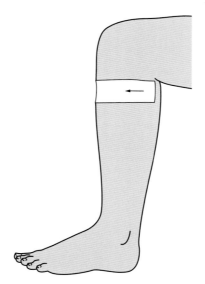

Tips

Easy to apply with the patient in the correct position, so the patient can be taught to do taping. This would allow the tape to be removed at night and reapplied in the morning, preventing the risk of an adverse skin reaction.

Chapter 7

Knee

CHAPTER CONTENTS

General knee and/or patellofemoral
pain   116
Patellar tendinosis   118
Knee support   120
Unload the fat pad   122
Knee support – Crystal Palace wrap   124
Knee support: alternative method – diamond
wrap   126

Sprain of the lateral collateral
ligament   128
Knee variation to reinforce the previous
basic tape job   130
Anterior cruciate taping   132
Continuous figure-of-eight wrap for the
knee   134
Unstable knee   136

General knee and/or patellofemoral pain

W.A. Hing and D.A. Reid

INDICATION

Taping for tibial rotation: limited painful knee flexion, due to a positional fault, in which tibial internal rotation mobilizations with movements (MWMs) have been painfree, and range has been increased.

Patients who have not responded to conventional patellofemoral glide taping (i.e. McConnell) may benefit from this type of taping.

FUNCTION

Taping corrects a positional fault throughout the patient's normal knee flexion/extension activities.

Internally rotating the tibia has been suggested to alter the tracking of the patella in the femoral groove.

MATERIAL

Spray adhesive or hypoallergenic undertape (Fixomull or Mefix). 38-mm strapping tape, shaver.

POSITION

Patient standing with knee in 5–10° of knee flexion. The patient then inverts the foot and internally rotates the tibia as far as possible on the femur. That is, the patient internally rotates the lower leg and turns the foot inwards while simultaneously externally rotating the femur and pointing the kneecap outwards (Fig. 7.1).

APPLICATION

Steps

1. Tape is started obliquely on the lateral aspect of the upper third of the leg (Fig. 7.2).

2. In an anterosuperior direction, wrap the tape diagonally around the anterior aspect of the knee joint.

3. Cross the medial aspect of the knee joint and run posteriorly across the back of the knee (Fig. 7.3).

4. Finally, secure to the lower third of the medial aspect of the thigh.

CHECK FUNCTION

Assess original painful movements (i.e. knee flexion). Ensure that knee flexion is painfree with the tape, and those aggravating activities can be performed with a reduction in symptoms.

CONTRAINDICATION

If taping causes changes or an increase in pain. Tape should not be left on for >48 h, and should be removed at any hint of skin irritation.

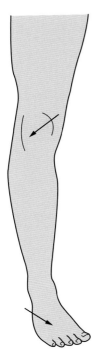

Figure 7.1

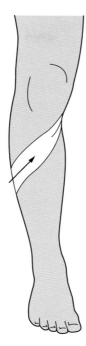

Figure 7.2

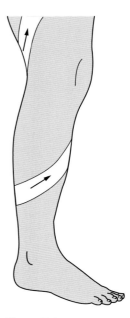

Figure 7.3

Tips

Safety permitting, you may find this easier with the patient standing on a plinth, so the patient's knee is not so far down. The patient may like to balance with the aid of a nearby wall.

Patellar tendinosis

W.A. Hing and D.A. Reid

INDICATION	Patellar tendinosis, unloading tendon or fat pad, also useful for managing the pain of Osgood–Schlatter's disease.
FUNCTION	Unload tendon and reduce pain in tendon or attachment.
MATERIALS	Spray adhesive or hypoallergenic undertape (Fixomull or Mefix). 38-mm strapping tape.
POSITION	Patient sitting with knee in full extension.

APPLICATION

Steps

1. Place one anchor strap over the thigh just above the superior patellar pole.

2. Attach one strip of tape to the anchor on the medial side of the knee, and pull the tape obliquely downward to the lateral side with the top edge of the tape passing just under the inferior patellar pole.

3. Repeat this action from lateral to medial, to make a cross-over effect, with the V of the cross in the midline just under the inferior patellar pole (Fig. 7.4).

4. Repeat this process until you have done two to three overlapping layers.

5. Do one final lock-off anchor over the top of the original anchor.

CHECK FUNCTION

When the patient stands and tries to bend the knee, there should be sufficient tension for the pressure to be felt over the tendon immediately under the kneecap.

Figure 7.4

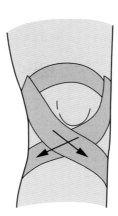

Tips

Use Mylanta (this is a stomach antacid which neutralizes the acidity of the tape: use extra strength) on the skin to avoid an adverse skin reaction to the tape. Before applying the tape, brush off the surface powder that appears when the Mylanta dries.

Knee support

G. Lapenskie

INDICATION	Retropatellar pain:

- patellofemoral dysfunction
- jumper's knee.

FUNCTION Purported to affect the angle of pull of the quadriceps muscle. Purported to affect the patellofemoral contact surface. May change the stress distribution pattern through the patellar tendon.

MATERIAL 10-cm cohesive bandage.

POSITION Sit the athlete on the edge of the plinth with the distal part of the thigh extending beyond the plinth. Bring the knee to 40° from full extension and maintain the position passively by placing the athlete's foot on your thigh.

APPLICATION **Steps**

1. Position the cohesive on the front of the thigh with one-quarter of the cohesive over the top of the patella. Anchor the cohesive in place by circumferentially wrapping the cohesive around the thigh until it overlaps.

2. When the cohesive passes over the superior position of the patella, put a twist in the cohesive by turning it 180°. Depress the superior pole of the patella with the thumb of the opposite hand and place the twist in the cohesive above the superior part of the patella to maintain the position of the patella (Fig. 7.5). Continue wrapping the cohesive around the thigh, placing a twist in the tensor over the top of the superolateral aspect of the patella (Fig. 7.6) and the superomedial aspect in subsequent passes (Fig. 7.7a).

3. Anchor the twist in place by wrapping the remaining length of the cohesive around the thigh (Fig. 7.7b).

CHECK FUNCTION   The patient should be able to perform or run without pain.

CONTRAINDICATIONS   Acute patellofemoral syndrome or retropatellar crepitus.

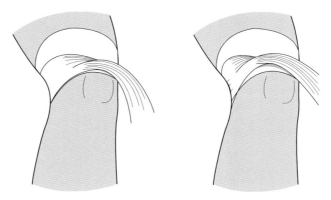

Figure 7.5   Figure 7.6

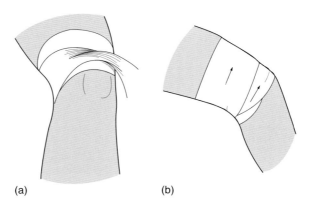

(a)   (b)

Figure 7.7

Unload the fat pad

J. McConnell

INDICATION	Inferior patellofemoral pain, hyperextended knees, irritated fat pad, post knee arthroscopy.
FUNCTION	Unloads irritated fat pad.
MATERIALS	Hypoallergenic tape (Endurafix/Fixomull/Hypafix/Mefix) and 3.8-cm tape.
POSITION	Patient lying, leg relaxed.

APPLICATION

Steps

Apply the hypoallergenic tape to the area to be taped.

1. Commence tape on the superior part of the patella to tip the inferior pole out of the fat pad (Fig. 7.8).
2. Next tape starts at the tibial tuberosity and goes out wide to the medial knee joint. The soft tissue is lifted towards the patella (Fig. 7.9).
3. The final tape starts at the tibial tuberosity, going wide to the lateral joint line.

CHECK FUNCTION	Check painful activity, which should now be painfree if the tape has been applied properly.
CONTRAINDICATION	Skin allergy – skin must be protected prior to taping.

Tips

The skin should have an orange-peel look.
The patient should be discouraged from hyperextending the knee.

Figure 7.8

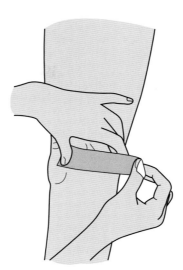

Figure 7.9

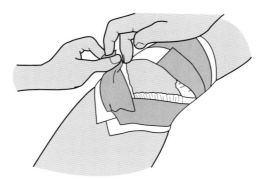

Knee support – Crystal Palace wrap

R. Macdonald

INDICATION	Retropatellar pain, jumper's knee and Osgood–Schlatter's disease.
FUNCTION	To relieve pressure of the patella on the femur. To relieve stress on the tibial tubercle.
MATERIALS	Gauze square, petroleum jelly, 5- or 7.5-cm stretch tape, 3.75-cm tape.
POSITION	Patient standing with the knee relaxed and slightly flexed.
APPLICATION	Cut a strip of stretch tape approximately 50 cm and place gauze in the centre.

Support strips

1. Lay tape on the back of the knee with the gauze square in the popliteal fossa. Mould the tape to the femoral condyles (Fig. 7.10).

2. Split the lateral strip into two tails. Stretch and twist tails separately and attach to the medial condyle, passing over the patellar tendon in the soft spot between the inferior patellar pole and tibial tubercle (Fig. 7.11). Repeat with the second tail (Fig. 7.12).

3. Stretch the medial strip across the twisted tails. Attach to the lateral condyle.

Lock strips

4. Close off with tape strips (Fig. 7.13).

CHECK FUNCTION	Have the patient squat. Is it tight in the popliteal fossa?
CONTRAINDICATIONS	Not suitable for those with rotated patellar dysfunction.

Tips

Best applied directly to the skin. Shave, wash and dry the skin. Apply skin prep or tough skin before taping.

Figure 7.10

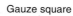
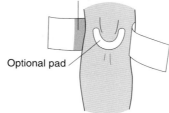

Gauze square

Optional pad

Figure 7.11

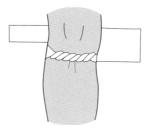

Figure 7.12

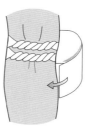

Figure 7.13

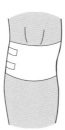

Knee support: alternative method – diamond wrap

R. Macdonald

APPLICATION Using 10-cm stretch tape (Fig. 7.10), apply as above. Split both ends of the tape, forming four tails (Fig. 7.14). Stretch the tails and apply firmly around the patella superiorly and inferiorly, interlocking the ends (Fig. 7.15). Close off with a strip of tape (Fig. 7.16).

Figure 7.14

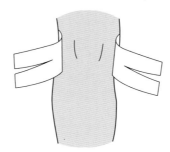

Figure 7.15

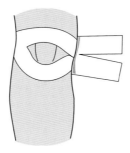

Figure 7.16

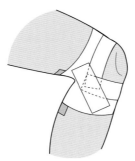

Sprain of the lateral collateral ligament

O. Rouillon

FUNCTION   To provide basic lateral stabilization of the knee.

MATERIALS   Lubricant, gauze squares, adhesive spray, two rolls of 6-cm stretch tape, 15-cm stretch tape, 3.8-cm tape.

POSITION   The patient is standing with the knee in 15° flexion and the roll of tape under the heel. The leg is pushed laterally. Apply the gauze with lubricant to the popliteal fossa; apply adhesive spray and prowrap.

APPLICATION   **Steps**

1. Using 6-cm stretch tape, apply two anchors to the lower third of the thigh and one anchor at the tibial tubercle (Fig. 7.17).

2. Using 6-cm stretch tape, apply a diagonal strip from the anteromedial aspect of the proximal anchor to the posteromedial aspect of the distal anchor.

3. The second symmetrical strip crosses the first at the centre of the medial joint line (Fig. 7.18).

4. Repeat this sequence with two more strips overlapping the previous strips by one-half anteriorly (Fig. 7.19).

5. Repeat the same sequence on the lateral knee joint.

6. Using six strips of 3.8-cm tape, apply a symmetrical montage, on top of the previous strips, with tension on the medial and lateral aspects of the knee joint (Fig. 7.20).

7. Lock the tape job in place with incomplete circles of tape (Fig. 7.21).

8. To protect the popliteal fossa, using a strip of 15-cm stretch tape, cut two tails on either end. Place the lubricated gauze square in the centre. Close the tails above and below the patellar poles (Fig. 7.22).

9. Finish with 6-cm stretch tape by reapplying the original anchors. Figure 7.23(a) shows the position of the leg for Figures 7.17 and 7.21, and Figure 7.23(b) shows the position of the leg for Figure 7.18.

CAUTION   Do not impinge the inferior patellar pole into fat pad.

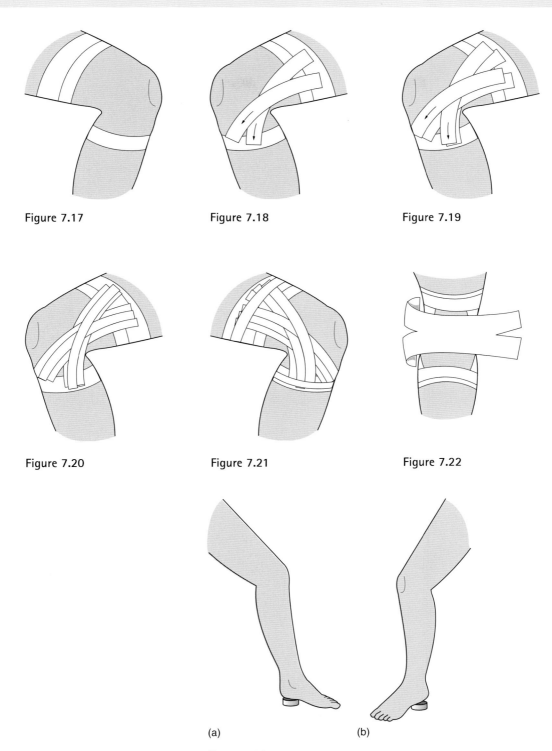

Figure 7.17

Figure 7.18

Figure 7.19

Figure 7.20

Figure 7.21

Figure 7.22

(a)

(b)

Figure 7.23

Knee variation to reinforce the previous basic tape job

O. Rouillon

INDICATIONS

To stabilize the tibia on the femur and support the anterior cruciate ligament.

FUNCTION

To stabilize anterior drawer; to limit medial/lateral rotation of femur or tibia; to limit hyperextension. To relieve stress at the attachment of the patellar tendon on the tibial tubercle.

MATERIALS

8-cm stretch tape, 3.8-cm tape.

POSITION

The knee is flexed with the heel on the tape roll and the leg in neutral position.

APPLICATION

Using 8-cm stretch tape, apply two anchors to the lower third of the thigh and one anchor distal to the tibial tubercle. Use one strip of 3.8-cm tape 25–30 cm long. Starting on the anterolateral aspect of the distal anchor, pass with full tension anteriorly across the tibial tubercle and diagonally upwards to the proximal anchor on the medial side. Apply a second strip on the opposite side with the same tension (Fig. 7.24).

Apply two more strips medially and laterally over the initial strips, superimposed on the inferior tails, and fanning out and overlapping by one-half, to attach to the proximal anchor (Figs 7.25 and 7.26). Lock these six strips in place with tape above and below without tension (Fig. 7.27a). Figure 7.27b shows the position of the leg for the taping procedure.

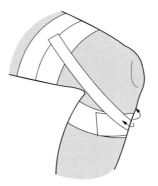

Figure 7.24

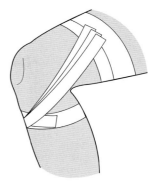

Figure 7.25

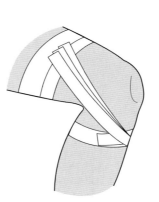

Figure 7.26

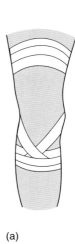

(a)

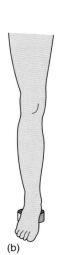

(b)

Figure 7.27

Anterior cruciate taping

K.E. Wright

INDICATION Sprain to the anterior cruciate ligament of the knee.

FUNCTION To provide support and stability to the knee's anterior cruciate ligament.

MATERIALS 3.8-cm adhesive tape, 7.5-cm elastic tape and gauze with lubricant.

POSITION Knee and hip joints should be positioned in slight flexion.

APPLICATION **Steps**

1. Apply gauze and lubricant to the posterior aspect of the knee joint. You should also apply an anchor strip of 7.5-cm elastic tape around the upper third of the thigh. Comment: in this pretaping procedure, do not compress the popliteal fossa.

2. Using 7.5-cm elastic tape, begin on the lower leg's lateral aspect, approximately 2.5 cm below the patella. Encircle the lower leg, move anteriorly, then medially, continuing to the posterior aspect and returning to the lateral side. Angle the tape below the patella, cross the medial joint line and popliteal fossa, and spiral up to the anterior portion of the upper thigh's anchor (Fig. 7.29).

3. The next strip of 7.5-cm elastic tape will begin on the anterior aspect of the proximal anchor (Fig. 7.30) and cross the thigh's medial portion, covering the popliteal fossa, encircling the lower leg and crossing the popliteal fossa again. You will finish by spiralling up to the anterior aspect of the thigh's proximal anchor (Fig. 7.31).

4. Repeat step 3.

5. Secure this technique by applying 3.8-cm adhesive tape over the thigh's anchor (Fig. 7.32).

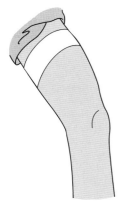

Figure 7.28

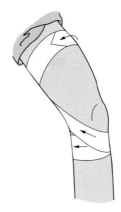

Figure 7.29

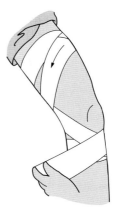

Figure 7.30

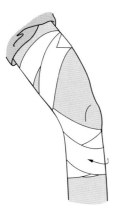

Figure 7.31

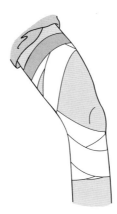

Figure 7.32

Continuous figure–of–eight wrap for the knee

K.E. Wright

INDICATION	Sprains to the knee joint.
FUNCTION	To provide support to the knee joint.
MATERIALS	10-cm elastic wrap, and 3.8-cm adhesive tape.
POSITION	Knee joint placed in slight flexion.
APPLICATION	**Steps**

1. Begin the wrap on the lateral/posterior aspect of the lower leg. Encircle the lower leg, moving medially to laterally.

2. Angle the wrap below the patella and cross the medial joint line (Fig. 7.33). Cover the thigh's posterior and lateral aspect. Encircle the thigh, moving medially to laterally (Fig. 7.34). Angle the wrap downward, staying above the patella, and crossing the medial joint line (Fig. 7.35). Cross the popliteal space and encircle the lower leg (Fig. 7.36).

3. Proceed with the wrap, crossing the lateral joint line and angling above the patella (Fig. 7.37). Encircle the thigh and, on the posterior aspect, angle across the knee's lateral joint line, staying below the patella (Fig. 7.38). This configuration should resemble a diamond shape around the patella and cover from mid-thigh to the gastrocnemius belly. Secure this wrap with 2.5-cm adhesive tape, applied at the wrap's loose end.

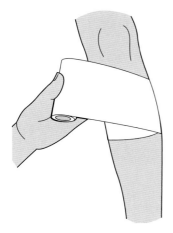

Figure 7.33

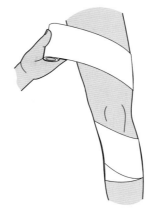

Figure 7.34

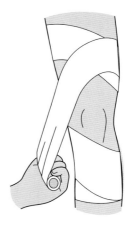

Figure 7.35

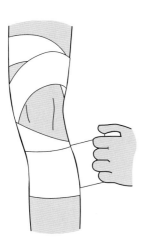

Figure 7.36

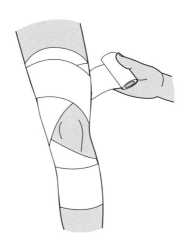

Figure 7.37

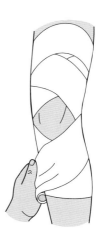

Figure 7.38

Unstable knee

A. DeBruyne

INDICATION

Unstable knee after light or moderate injury, elongation of anterior cruciate ligament (ACL), posterior cruciate ligament (PCL), light inflammation of patellar tendon, during rehabilitation after surgery.

FUNCTION

Range of motion protection for flexion/extension beyond 90°. Stabilization for light transitory ligament injury.

MATERIALS

Padding for popliteal fossa and tendons, 2.5-, 5-, 7.5-cm stretch tape and 2.5-cm rigid tape.

POSITION

Patient lying prone for the first part. Then supine with the knee in 60° flexion for the second part.

APPLICATION

Steps

- Place the pad on the back of the knee and anchor with two diagonal and one transverse strips of 5-cm stretch tape. These strips should cover the hamstring tendons as they will act as anchors for the anterior strips (Fig. 7.39).

- *Tibial stabilization anchor*: using 7.5-cm stretch, place across the front of the knee at the upper border, level with the centre of the patellar tendon. Proceed around the back of the knee, across the front again, to finish on the medial side.

- Using 2.5-cm stretch, construct a basketweave to duplicate the ACL and PCL attachments with four strips:
  1. The first strip starts over the the top of the patella and runs down close to the patella across the medial joint line to finish on the tibial anchor, duplicating the PCL (Fig. 7.40).
  2. Repeat on the lateral side.
  3. The next strip starts on the semitendinosis tendon and runs forward to cross the tibial tubercle, duplicating the ACL (Fig. 7.41).
  4. Repeat this strip, starting on the biceps femoris tendon and crossing the previous strip on the tibial tubercle.

Figure 7.39

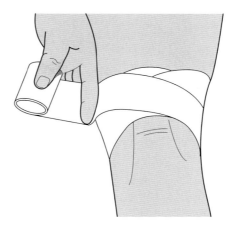

Figure 7.40

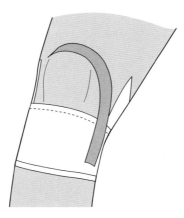

Figure 7.41

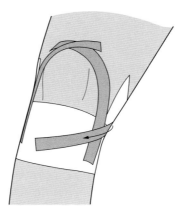

- Repeat this procedure three more times, moving proximally. The four strips cross each other over the medial and later joint lines (Figs 7.42 and 7.43).

- *Figure-of-eight stabilizing anchor*: using 7.5-cm stretch, start medially, run the tape up over the top of the patella, around the back of the knee, up over the patella again, to finish on the lateral side (Fig. 7.44).

- Reapply tibial stabilizing anchor, and close off the end with a piece of 2.5-cm tape.

- Manually stretch out the back of the knee if it is too tight.

CHECK FUNCTION

Let the athlete walk a few metres to see how it feels.

CONTRAINDICATION

All injuries that need surgery.

Tips

May reinforce the basketweave with rigid tape for greater stability.

Figure 7.42

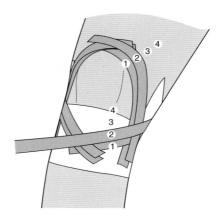

Figure 7.43

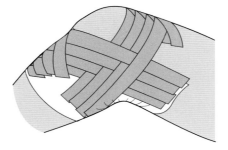

Figure 7.44

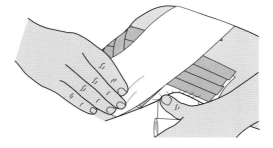

Chapter **8**

Lumbar spine

CHAPTER CONTENTS

Lumbar spine taping 142
Frontal plane pelvic stability 144

Sacroiliac joint 146
Chronic low-back and leg pain 148

Lumbar spine taping

W.A. Hing and D.A. Reid

INDICATION
Lumbar dysfunction and pain. Avoidance of painful lumbar flexion or postures.
Application following Mulligan lumbar sustained natural apophyseal glides (SNAGs) or McKenzie extensions.

FUNCTION
Maintains neutral to extended lumbar lordosis. Avoids pain-provoking positions and facilitates a more extended posture.

MATERIAL
Spray adhesive or hypoallergenic undertape (Fixomull or Mefix). 38-mm or 50-mm strapping tape.

POSITION
Patient lying prone or may be taped in sitting or standing.
Patient must be able to achieve a relaxed and painfree extended lumbar posture (lordosis) while the tape is being applied.

APPLICATION

Steps

1. Spine in neutral to slightly extended position with lumbar curvatures maintained.

2. Anchor strips are applied to the top and bottom of the area to be taped.

3. An X is formed across the lumbar region from the top anchor to the bottom anchor, with the centre of the X overlying L2–3 region (Fig. 8.1). Repeat this X with two more strips overlapping the previous strips by half.

4. The top and bottom of the X are then reanchored.

CHECK FUNCTION
Assess original painful movements (i.e. flexion, reaching forward). Movements should now be painfree and limited at end of range.

CONTRAINDICATION
Check skin reaction to tape and tell the patient to remove it if an adverse skin reaction occurs. Tape should not be left on for more than 48 h.

Figure 8.1

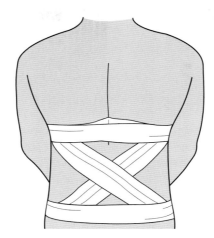

Tips

This procedure is easy to apply with the patient in the correct position, so a family member could be taught to do the taping. This would allow the tape to be removed at night and reapplied in the morning, preventing the risk of an adverse skin reaction.

Frontal plane pelvic stability

A. Hughes

INDICATION   Conditions aggravated by excessive lateral horizontal pelvic tilt, trochanteric bursitis, piriformis syndrome, sacroiliac joint (SIJ) instability, iliotibial band (ITB) friction syndrome or runner's knee, patellofemoral pain.

FUNCTION   To control excessive lateral horizontal pelvic tilt (Trendelenberg sign) and facilitate femoral external rotation to limit lateral and posterior displacement of the femoral greater trochanter in stance phase.

MATERIAL   3.8-cm rigid tape, 5-cm Fixomull or Hypafix hypoallergenic tape.

POSITION   Standing with the feet slightly apart and 20° externally rotated. Hands crossed over the shoulders, and thoracic spine rotated away from the side to be taped.

APPLICATION   **Steps**

Apply the hypoallergenic tape in the same sequence as the rigid tape, as follows:

1. Apply a continuous strip of rigid tape from the anteromedial aspect of the lower third of the thigh, moving superolaterally, behind the greater trochanter, over the SIJ to finish on the contralateral side of the low lumbar spine (Fig. 8.2).

2. Increase tension when passing over the posterolateral aspect, by creating skin folds with the therapist's other hand. This is done by pinching the soft tissue and moving it in the direction opposite to the tape application (Figs. 8.3 and 8.4).

3. Apply two closing locks with Fixomull to either end of the tape (Fig. 8.5).

CHECK FUNCTION   Ask the patient to resume a single-leg stance. The technique should neutralize any Trendelenberg sign.

CONTRAINDICATION   Ensure that the rigid tape does not extend beyond the hypoallergenic tape, thus avoiding possible skin irritation. Avoid using rigid tape with older patients.

Figure 8.2

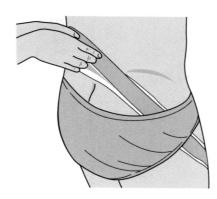

Figure 8.3

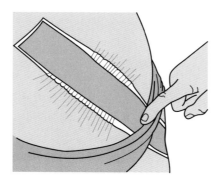

Figure 8.4

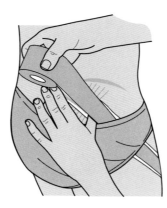

Figure 8.5

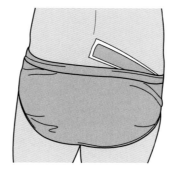

Sacroiliac joint

W.A. Hing and D.A. Reid

INDICATION

Pain with weight-bearing and walking. Diagnosed SIJ dysfunction which responds to Mulligan mobilization with movement (MWM). Patients may complain of leg pain mimicking a disc, but with normal straight-leg raise (SLR). Also with positive active straight-leg-raise test (Vleeming).

FUNCTION

Taping corrects the positional fault, by holding the ilium in its correct position on the sacrum.

In general, there are two positional faults: (1) anterior innominate, where the ilium will be *glided* posterior to the sacrum; and (2) posterior innominate, where the ilium will be *glided* anterior to the sacrum.

MATERIAL

Spray adhesive or hypoallergenic undertape (Fixomull or Mefix). 38-mm strapping tape.

POSITION

If taping for an anterior innominate – patient in prone lying.

APPLICATION

Steps

1. Taping for anterior innonimate – pain with McKenzie extension in lying (Fig. 8.6).

2. Begin with the tape on front of the anterior superior iliac spine (Fig. 8.7).

3. Wrap tape obliquely and superiorly to terminate over the lumbar spine (Fig. 8.7).

4. Secure with a second piece of tape (Fig. 8.8).

CHECK FUNCTION

Assess original painful movements (i.e. extension in lying, extension in standing, flexion in standing). Movements should now have painfree full range of motion and function.

CONTRAINDICATION

If taping causes changes or an increase in pain. Tape should not be left on for >48 h, and should be removed at any hint of skin irritation.

Figure 8.6

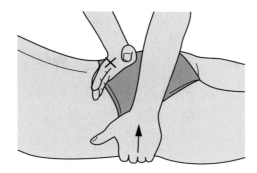

Figure 8.7

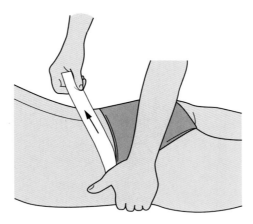

Figure 8.8

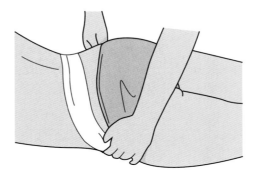

 Tips

If the patient has pain with gait, try walking behind the patient, manually applying the MWM posterior glide to the ilium. If this is successful, taping should have positive results.

Chronic low–back and leg pain

J. McConnell

INDICATION	Nerve root irritation.
FUNCTION	Unloads irritated neural and fascial tissue.
MATERIAL	Hypoallergenic tape (Endurafix/Fixomull/Hypafix/Mefix) and 3.8-cm tape.
POSITION	Patient standing.

APPLICATION

Steps

Apply the hypoallergenic tape to the area to be taped:

1. Anchor first tape at ischium and follow gluteal fold proximal to greater trochanter, lifting soft tissue proximally (Fig. 8.9).

2. Second tape is parallel to the natal cleft with the skin lifted towards the buttock (Fig. 8.10).

3. Third tape joins the first and second tapes and runs lateral to medial (Fig. 8.10).

4. The tape then follows the appropriate nerve root and is placed at a diagonal, first on the upper leg and then on the lower leg, with the skin being lifted towards the head each time (Fig. 8.11).

CHECK FUNCTION	Check painful activity, which should now be painfree if the tape has been applied properly.
CONTRAINDICATION	Skin allergy – skin must be protected before taping.

Tips

The symptoms may intensify slightly distally, but as soon as the distal tape is in situ, the symptoms minimize.

Figure 8.9

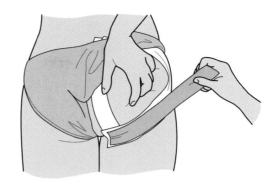

Figure 8.10

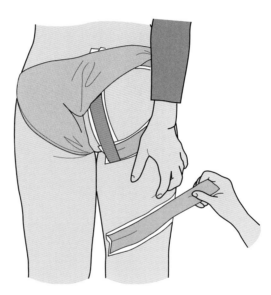

Figure 8.11

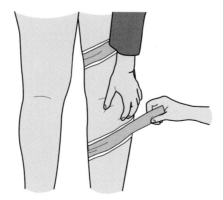

Chapter **9**

Thoracic spine

CHAPTER CONTENTS

Thoracic spine taping   152
Thoracic spine unload   154
Winging scapulae   156

Scapular control – Watson's strap   158
Scapular retraction   160

Thoracic spine taping

W.A. Hing and D.A. Reid

INDICATION	Thoracic pain and posture correction. Neck pain associated with cervical end-range rotation or neck retraction. Application following Mulligan sustained natural apophyseal glides (SNAGs) to cervico-thoracic or thoracic spine.
FUNCTION	Maintains neutral to retracted thoracic posture, and avoids pain-provoking postures. Decreases pain during specific neck movements (end-range cervical rotation or retraction, by holding shoulder girdle into a more retracted position).
MATERIALS	Spray adhesive or hypoallergenic undertape (Fixomull or Mefix). 38-mm or 50-mm strapping tape.
POSITION	Patient sitting with shoulders retracted.
APPLICATION	**Steps**

1. Place a single horizontal strip of tape across the shoulder blades of the patient, taping the scapulae into a mid-range, retracted position (Fig. 9.1).

2. The tape should lie just under the spine of the scapulae, running from lateral border to lateral border of each shoulder blade.

3. Place a second piece of tape over the initial taping.

CHECK FUNCTION	Assess original painful movements (i.e. cervical rotation or arm function and ability to reach). Movements should now be painfree and limited at end of range.
CONTRAINDICATION	If taping causes changes or an increase in pain. Tape should not be left on for >48 h, and should be removed at any hint of skin irritation. If there is a potential for tape reaction, use hypoallergenic undertape such as Fixomull.

Figure 9.1

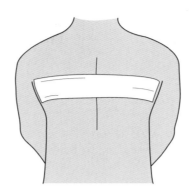

Tips

This procedure is easy to apply with the patient in the correct position, so a family member could be taught to do taping. This would allow the tape to be removed at night and reapplied in the morning, preventing the risk of an adverse skin reaction.

Thoracic spine unload

D. Kneeshaw

INDICATION	Thoracic facet sprain. Overuse thoracic paraspinal muscles.
FUNCTION	To support specific vertebrae and reduce muscle activity at that vertebral level.
MATERIALS	Hypoallergenic tape (Fixomull or Mefix). 4.0-cm rigid strapping tape.
POSITION	Neutral scapula posture.
APPLICATION	**Steps** 1. Using hypoallergenic tape, lay the tape down to form a small square surrounding the offending vertebrae, to about one vertebra above and below. 2. Using rigid tape, attach one end of the tape to a corner of the square and lay the tape to the adjacent corner, shortening the tissue to create a puckering effect (Fig. 9.2). 3. Repeat the previous procedure for each side of the square.
CONTRAINDICATION	Patients with a history of hypersensitive skin.

Tips

- The exposed tissue in the centre of the square should have an orange-peel appearance.

- Useful for acute, painful conditions that have an associated muscular spasm.

Figure 9.2

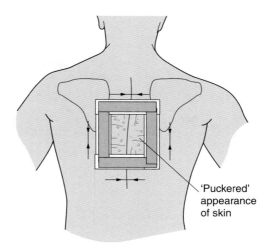

'Puckered'
appearance
of skin

Winging scapulae

D. Kneeshaw

INDICATION	Instability, impingement, tendinitis.
FUNCTION	To reposition the scapulae to a neutral posture and allow proper activation of serratus anterior and lower trapezius.
MATERIALS	Hypoallergenic tape (Fixomull or Mefix). 4.0-cm rigid strapping tape.
POSITION	Retracted and depressed scapular posture.

APPLICATION

Steps

1. Using hypoallergenic tape, form an overlapping row of three to four straps from just lateral of the medial border (central) of one scapula to the other.

2. Using rigid tape, apply over the hypoallergenic tape with firm pressure to reinforce the retracted and depressed scapular posture (Fig. 9.3).

CHECK FUNCTION

- Assess scapulo-humeral rhythm.
- Assess amount of winging by attempting to push your index finger under the inferior angle of the scapula – only one phalange should be concealed.

CONTRAINDICATION Patients with a history of hypersensitive skin.

Figure 9.3

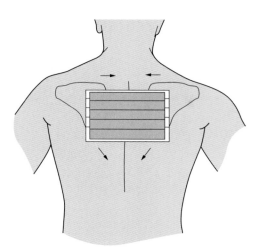

Scapular control – Watson's strap

D. Kneeshaw

INDICATION	Impingement, tendinitis.
FUNCTION	To reposition the scapulae in a neutral position and allow proper activation of the rhomboids and trapezius muscles.
MATERIALS	Hypoallergenic tape (Fixomull or Mefix). 4.0-cm rigid strapping tape.
POSITION	Neutral scapular posture.

APPLICATION

Steps

1. Lay the hypoallergenic tape from the axilla, across the middle third of the scapula, to the mid-point of the spine of the contralateral scapula.

2. Using rigid tape, begin at the axilla and apply no pressure until the tape meets the lateral border of the scapula.

3. The therapist then places one hand in the axilla and applies a superomedial pressure to the scapula, thus resulting in a lateral rotation movement (Fig. 9.4).

4. Simultaneously apply the tape to the mid-point of the spine of the contralateral scapula.

CHECK FUNCTION

- Assess scapulo-humeral rhythm in abduction and forward flexion.
- Assess pain levels compared with before.

CONTRAINDICATION

Patients with a history of hypersensitive skin.

Tips

- Ask hirsute individuals to shave their armpits 48 h before tape application.

Figure 9.4

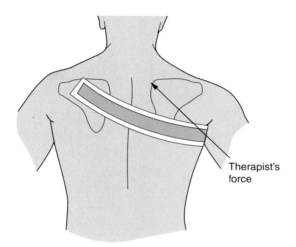

Therapist's
force

Scapular retraction

D. Kneeshaw

INDICATION	Instability, impingement, tendinitis.
FUNCTION	Reposition the scapular to a neutral posture and shorten the rhomboids, lower trapezius or serratus anterior.
MATERIALS	Hypoallergenic tape (Fixomull or Mefix). 4.0-cm rigid strapping tape.
POSITION	Scapulae in retracted, depressed posture.
APPLICATION	**Steps**

1. Using hypoallergenic tape, lay the tape from the coracoid process posteriorly across the lateral aspect of the acromion to a point just lateral to the T7 spinous process.
2. Using rigid tape, lay over the hypoallergenic tape – without pressure – to the posterior aspect of the shoulder and finally apply a firm pressure medially to position the scapula in a retracted, depressed posture (Fig. 9.5).

CONTRAINDICATION	Patients with a history of hypersensitive skin.

Figure 9.5

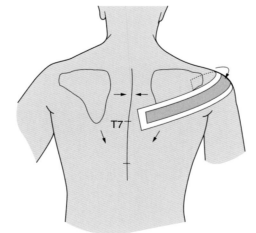

Tips

- Do not over-retract or depress the scapulae.

Chapter **10**

Shoulder girdle

CHAPTER CONTENTS

Subluxation of acromioclavicular joint   162
Acromioclavicular joint strap   164
Acromioclavicular joint taping   166
Acromioclavicular taping for sport using
   stretch tape   170

Anterior instability – Rigney's strap   174
Relocation of the humeral head   176
Impingement syndrome (Allingham's
   strap)   178
Multidirectional instability   180
Overactive upper trapezius   182

Subluxation of acromioclavicular joint

W.A. Hing and D.A. Reid

INDICATION
Disruption of the acromioclavicular (AC) joint complex grades 1 and 2.

FUNCTION
To provide a degree of support to stretched ligaments.

MATERIALS
Spray adhesive or hypoallergenic undertape (Fixomull or Mefix). 38-mm strapping tape, 38-mm elastic adhesive bandage (EAB).

POSITION
Patient sitting with the hand on the hip or, alternatively, rest the elbow on a table so the arm sits at about 45° away from the side.

APPLICATION

Steps

1. Apply a piece of hypoallergenic undertape (Fixomull) as an anchor from the front of the chest over the end of the clavicle to the shoulder blade.

2. Attach a length of tape from the anchor down the front of the arm, around the elbow and back up the other side of the arm to the anchor on the shoulder blade (Fig. 10.1).

3. Next, apply an EAB in the same fashion. (Adhesive tape can also be used.)

4. Apply an EAB anchor around the arm just above the biceps muscle. Ensure that it is not too tight to compromise the circulation (Fig. 10.2). Re-apply anchor over AC joint.

5. Once this is secure, cut off the tape which has been previously applied around the elbow (Fig. 10.3). Removing this originally applied piece of tape allows more freedom of movement for the arm. The reason for originally applying it was to create enough tension on the AC joint to keep it down. They often pop up when damaged.

CONTRAINDICATION
Grade 3 injury will probably need orthopaedic review.

Figure 10.1

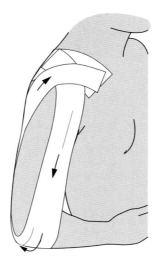

Figure 10.2

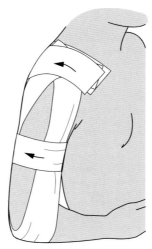

Figure 10.3

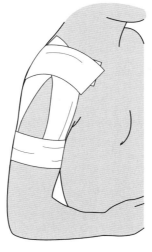

Acromioclavicular joint strap

D. Kneeshaw

INDICATION	Ligamentous sprain about the AC joint.
FUNCTION	To reduce superior migration of the clavicle and allow proper rotation and translation of the joint.
MATERIALS	± Hypoallergenic tape (Fixomull or Mefix). 4.0-cm rigid strapping tape.
POSITION	Arm by the side in neutral posture.

APPLICATION

Steps

1. Using hypoallergenic tape, lay the tape from around mid-height pectoralis major, superior to the nipple, to the inferior angle of the scapula (Fig. 10.4).

2. Using rigid tape, lay the tape from anterior to posterior with firm pressure in an inferior direction, on the posterior side. Do not apply posterior force, only inferior.

CHECK FUNCTION

1. Assess the amount of AC joint elevation in horizontal flexion and forward flexion.

2. Assess pain levels compared with before.

CONTRAINDICATION

Patients with a history of hypersensitive skin.

Figure 10.4

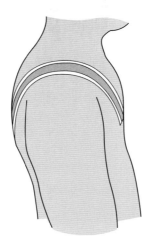

Acromioclavicular joint taping

A. Hughes

INDICATION Acute distraction of the AC joint (grade 1–3 ligamentous injuries). May be modified for gleno-humeral joint instability.

FUNCTION To relieve superior shoulder pain by: (1) maintaining approximation of the acromion and distal end of the clavicle following AC joint injury; (2) assisting in depressing the distal end of the clavicle.

MATERIALS 5-cm hypoallergenic pretape (Fixomull/Hypafix), 3.8-cm rigid tape and 10-cm elastic adhesive tape.

POSITION Sitting with the arm supported and abducted 50–60° to the horizontal, and 10° horizontal flexion.

APPLICATION **Steps**

1. Apply the Fixomull tape in the same sequence as the rigid tape which follows, and ensure that the rigid tape does not extend beyond the border of the Fixomull as skin reaction is likely to occur in this area of the body.

2. Apply two strips of rigid tape from below the inferior angle of the scapula, over the shoulder (avoiding the AC joint) to the subpectoral region. Pull down on the clavicle and gather up the pectoral soft tissues prior to attaching (Fig. 10.5).

3. Apply one to two incomplete anchors to the humerus distal to the deltoid insertion, overlapping by two-thirds.

4. Attach two support strips from the anterior and posterior aspects of the humeral anchors. Passing, in a supero-posterior and supero-anterior direction, attach to the posterior and anterior aspects of the thoracic anchor respectively. Repeat with two more support strips, overlapping the previous strips by two-thirds (Fig. 10.6).

5. Reapply the original anchors on the humerus.

6. Apply two locking anchors to the thorax with either Fixomull or an elastic adhesive tape, to ensure the thoracic tapes do not lift during arm elevation (Figs 10.7 and 10.8).

Figure 10.5

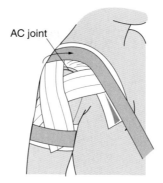

AC joint

Figure 10.6

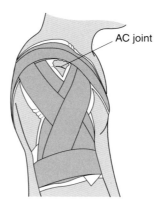

AC joint

Figure 10.7

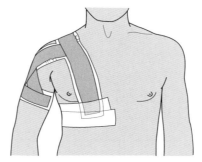

Figure 10.8

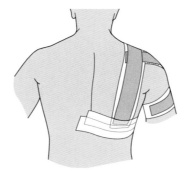

CHECK FUNCTION

In a standing position, the affected arm should be maintained in approximately 10° of abduction.

Note the freedom of motion available into elevation (Fig. 10.9).

CONTRAINDICATION

Avoid using rigid tape with older patients as skin reaction may occur. In this case, the complete technique may be applied with hypoallergenic tape such as Fixomull/Hypafix.

Tips

Adapt the technique for gleno-humeral joint instabilities by applying the humeral cross-over tapes (Fig. 10.6) to cover a greater area of the anterior gleno-humeral joint (limiting horizontal extension) or, to the posterior gleno-humeral joint (limiting horizontal flexion). This will also restrict elevation of the arm.

The AC joint is not covered by tape with this technique (Figs 10.5–10.7). It is therefore possible to use therapeutic agents whilst the tape is in place.

Figure 10.9

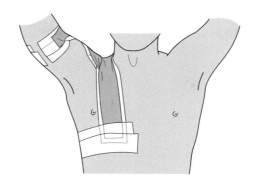

Acromioclavicular taping for sport using stretch tape

O. Rouillon

INDICATIONS
- Return to sport after AC subluxation
- preventive for athletes with residual after-effects
- for sprains where rigid tape is not necessary.

FUNCTION   To control the clavicle actively and passively during sport.

MATERIALS   Lubricant, three to four gauze squares, one to two rolls of 6-cm stretch tape, 10-cm cohesive bandage.

POSITION   Sitting with the arm abducted 80°.

APPLICATION   Protect the nipple with lubricant and pad. Protect the AC joint with lubricant and pad.
Place an anchor of 6-cm stretch tape around the upper arm in the V of the deltoid without tension. Place a semicircular anchor around the thorax (Fig. 10.10).

Support strips
1. Using 6-cm stretch tape, start the first strip at the sternoclavicular joint and pull with moderate tension over the AC joint to finish on the posterior aspect of the arm anchor (Fig. 10.11).

2. The second strip starts at the base of the neck posteriorly and crosses the AC joint, finishing on the anterior aspect of the arm anchor (Fig. 10.12).

3. The third strip starts on the thoracic vertebra, crosses the AC joint and finishes on the arm anchor anterior to strip 2 (Fig. 10.13).

Figure 10.10

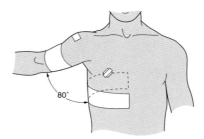

Figure 10.11

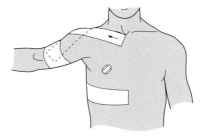

Figure 10.12

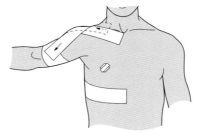

Figure 10.13

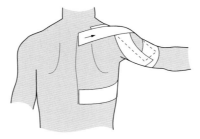

Three more strips are applied (with 6-cm tape):

1. The first strip passes from the posterior thoracic anchor over the AC joint, to finish on the anterior thoracic anchor in the sagittal plane (Fig. 10.14).

2. The second strip starts at a 30° angle to the first and crosses the first strip at the AC joint.

3. The third strip is symmetrical to the second and crosses the previous two strips at the AC joint (Fig. 10.15).

Anchors (locking strips)

Using 6-cm stretch tape, repeat the initial anchors around the arm and thorax (Fig. 10.16).

To maintain the tape job in place, apply a 10-cm cohesive bandage a couple of times around the thorax.

CHECK FUNCTION

- Test the active range of motion.

- Check if the tape job is supportive.

Figure 10.14

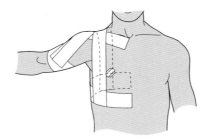

Figure 10.15

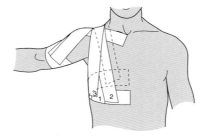

Figure 10.16

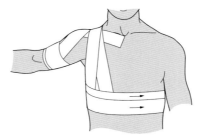

Anterior instability – Rigney's strap

D. Kneeshaw

INDICATION	Anterior instability.
FUNCTION	To reduce available external rotation of the gleno-humeral joint in positions of abduction and scaption.
MATERIALS	5.0-cm stretch tape, 4.0-cm rigid strapping tape.
POSITION	Affected shoulder in 90° abduction, full internal rotation, and elbow at 90° with hand resting on plinth.

APPLICATION

Steps

1. Anchors: using stretch tape, place one anchor around the distal portion of the upper arm, proximal to the elbow. Place a second around the thorax, below the extent of the pectoral muscles. Add a heel-and-lace pad or gauze over the nipple for protection (Fig. 10.17).

2. Supports: using rigid tape, start on the arm anchor posteromedially and continue along the posterior aspect of the shoulder, crossing the superior aspect of the shoulder, finishing on the chest anchor.

3. Repeat several times in an overlapping fashion.

4. Reapply the original anchors.

CONTRAINDICATION Patients with a history of hypersensitive skin.

Tips

- Note that for some overhead sports requiring a larger 'cock-up' phase (e.g. throwing), this tape does hinder performance.

- It is most effective for contact sports such as rugby.

Figure 10.17

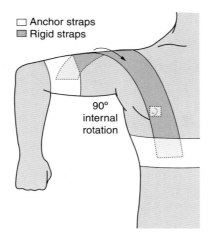

☐ Anchor straps
▨ Rigid straps

90°
internal
rotation

Relocation of the humeral head

J. McConnell

INDICATION

Anterior shoulder instability, impingement problems, rotator cuff tears and adhesive capsulitis.

FUNCTION

Taping corrects the positional fault by lifting the anterior aspect of the humeral head up and back, to increase the space between the humeral head and the acromium.

MATERIALS

Hypoallergenic tape (Endurafix/Fixomull/Hypafix/Mefix) and 3.8-cm tape.

POSITION

Patient standing or sitting on chair or stool, arms resting by the side.

APPLICATION

Steps

Apply the hypoallergenic tape to the area to be taped.

1. Anchor a strip of tape on the anterior aspect of the glenohumeral joint.

2. With the thumb of the other hand, lift the head of the humerus up and back (Fig. 10.18).

3. Firmly pull the tape diagonally across the scapula, to finish just medial to the inferior border of the scapula.

Care must be taken not to pull too hard on the skin anteriorly, as the skin is sensitive in this region and may break down if not looked after properly.

CHECK FUNCTION

Check painful activity, which should now be painfree if the tape has been applied properly.

CONTRAINDICATION

Skin allergy – skin must be protected before taping.

Figure 10.18

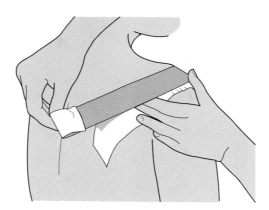

 Tips

To ensure long-term reductions in symptoms, work on improving thoracic spine mobility and muscle training of the scapular and glenohumeral stabilizers.

Impingement syndrome (Allingham's strap)

D. Kneeshaw

INDICATION	Impingement syndrome of the rotator cuff insertion under the acromion.
FUNCTION	To improve the actions of the shoulder stabilizers. To reduce the superior translation of the humeral head on the glenoid fossa.
MATERIALS	Hypoallergenic tape (Fixomull or Mefix). 3.8-cm rigid strapping tape.
POSITION	Seated with the arm by the side in neutral posture.

APPLICATION

Steps

Cover the area to be taped with the hypoallergenic tape in the same sequence as the rigid tape to follow.

1. Start from the middle deltoid insertion and lay the tape down to just before the acromion.
2. Then, pull firmly to a point halfway between the neck and shoulder on the upper trapezius fibres.
3. Repeat with a second strip, starting from the anterior aspect of deltoid, overlapping the first, and finishing at the same point (Fig. 10.19).
4. Repeat with a third strip, starting from the posterior aspect of deltoid and continuing as above.

CHECK FUNCTION

- Assess the amount of hitching through abduction.
- Assess pain levels compared with before.

CONTRAINDICATION   Patients with a history of hypersensitive skin.

Figure 10.19

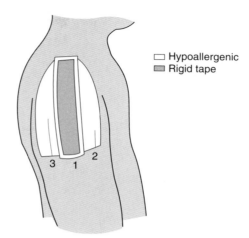

☐ Hypoallergenic
▨ Rigid tape

Tips

Purported to be most effective in the acute stage of impingement.

Multidirectional instability

J. McConnell

INDICATION	Multidirectional shoulder instability.
FUNCTION	Taping stabilizes the head of humerus in the glenoid cavity.
MATERIALS	Hypoallergenic tape (Endurafix/Fixomull/Hypafix/Mefix) and 3.8-cm tape.
POSITION	Patient sitting on chair or stool, forearm supported on table at 30° of scaption.

APPLICATION

Steps

Apply the hypoallergenic tape to the area to be taped.

1. Anchor the first piece of tape over the middle deltoid and lift the head of the humerus up.

2. The second piece commences anteriorly on the humerus and passes in a diagonal over the clavicle and anchors on the spine of the scapula. The humerus again is lifted superiorly (Fig. 10.20).

3. The third piece of tape is commenced on the posterior deltoid and runs along the spine of the scapula to the nape of the neck. The humerus is lifted superiorly. This piece gives the patient some posterior stability. Without this piece of tape the patient often feels insecure.

CHECK FUNCTION

Check painful activity, which should now be painfree if the tape has been applied properly.

CONTRAINDICATION

Skin allergy – skin must be protected before taping.

Tips

Initially work on training the deltoid muscle as a stabilizer.

Figure 10.20

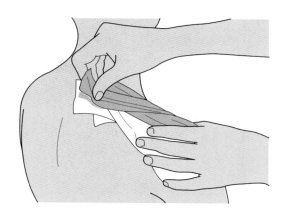

Overactive upper trapezius

D. Kneeshaw

INDICATION	Variety of neck and shoulder conditions that result in, or are exacerbated by, hitching of the shoulder.
FUNCTION	To bunch the upper trapezius fibres laterally, thereby reducing their ability to activate, which in turn, results in reduced hitching.
MATERIALS	Hypoallergenic tape (Fixomull or Mefix). 4.0-cm rigid strapping tape.
POSITION	Neutral scapular posture.

APPLICATION

Steps

1. Using hypoallergenic tape, lay the tape from a point at the level of T7, medial to the medial border of the scapula.

2. Using rigid tape, apply over the hypoallergenic tape, with a posterior-inferior force, to bunch the upper trapezius fibres (Fig. 10.21).

3. Continue this pressure as the rest of the tape is laid down.

CONTRAINDICATION Patient history of hypersensitive skin.

Figure 10.21

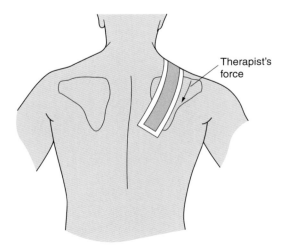

Therapist's force

Chapter **11**

Elbow, wrist and hand

CHAPTER CONTENTS

Tennis elbow (lateral epicondylosis)   184
Simple epicondylitis technique   186
Elbow hyperextension sprain   188
Prophylactic wrist taping   190
Wrist taping   192
Wrist taping   194

Inferior radioulnar joint taping   196
Contusion to the hand   198
Palm protective taping
   (the Russell web)   200
Protection of the metacarpophalangeal
   joints for boxers   204

Tennis elbow (lateral epicondylosis)

W.A. Hing and D.A. Reid

INDICATION	Lateral epicondyle pain
FUNCTION	To reduce the loading on the extensor mechanism, especially in movements of the forearm and wrist involving gripping and pronation.
MATERIALS	Spray adhesive or hypoallergenic undertape (Fixomull or Mefix). 38-mm strapping tape, shaver.
POSITION	Patient sitting or standing with the elbow flexed to 90° and the forearm fully supinated.

APPLICATION

Steps

1. Place an anchor midway around the forearm (Fig. 11.1).
2. With the arm in the above position, attach a strip of tape to the anchor on the medial side of the forearm. Direct it obliquely up the arm to slightly above the lateral epicondyle. Continue the tape around the lateral part of triceps and finish on the medial aspect of biceps (Fig. 11.2).
3. Apply a second strip of tape, following the same lines and overlapping the first strip by a third, usually in a more lateral direction (Fig. 11.3).
4. Reapply the first anchor.

CHECK FUNCTION   Once complete, the patient should feel the tape restrict the movements of elbow extension and pronation.

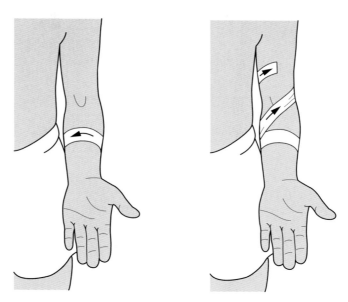

Figure 11.1   Figure 11.2

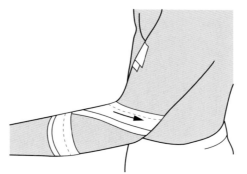

Figure 11.3

Simple epicondylitis technique

R. Macdonald

INDICATION	Tennis elbow – inflammation at the origin of the extensor tendons.
FUNCTION	To relieve stress on the origin of the tendon attachments. To realign the pull of the extensor tendons.
MATERIALS	3.8-cm tape (with strong adhesive mass), 5-cm cohesive bandage.
POSITION	Standing and facing operator with pronated arm resting on chair back.

APPLICATION

Steps

1. Visually observe the contracted belly of extensor carpi radialis brevis muscle, by applying resistance to the patient's extension of the third and fourth finger and wrist.

2. The patient flexes the elbow 90° across the chest to rest lightly on the opposite forearm. Take a strip of tape 10–15 cm long.

3. Stick tape to midline (palmar aspect) of the forearm just distal to the elbow crease, and spiral it superolaterally over the lateral epicondyle, to the olecranon/postero-inferior aspect of the humerus (Fig. 11.4).

4. Before attaching the tape, place the thumb of your other hand under the belly of the muscle and draw the tape firmly across the soft tissues to form a fold (Fig. 11.5).

5. Repeat this strip once more proximally, if necessary.

Hold in place with one or two turns of a cohesive bandage in a figure-of-eight pattern.

CHECK FUNCTION Ask the patient to make a fist to see if the technique is supportive, and relieves stress on the epicondyle.

Figure 11.4

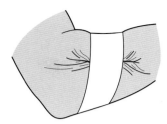

Figure 11.5

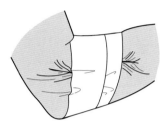

 Tips

Teach the technique to a friend or family member, as it is easy to apply.

Elbow hyperextension sprain

R. Macdonald

INDICATION	Elbow hyperextension, impingement, sprained medial collateral ligament.
FUNCTION	To limit the degree of elbow extension.
MATERIALS	Adhesive spray, gauze square, 7.5-cm stretch tape, 3.8-cm and 2.5-cm tape, 5-cm cohesive bandage.
POSITION	Standing, facing operator with the supinated flexed forearm resting on the back of the chair (with the fist clenched for application of anchors).
APPLICATION	**Steps**

Spray the arm, and apply a lubricated gauze square to the cubital fossa. Apply an anchor of stretch tape around the belly of biceps (contracted), and another around the proximal third of the forearm.

1. Flex elbow 45–60°, measure the distance between the upper and lower anchors.

2. Taking five strips of 2.5-cm tape (this length), construct a check rein (fan) on the table (Fig. 11.6).

3. Apply one end of the fan to the distal anchor and secure it in place with two or three strips of tape on front of the arm only. Before attaching the other end to the proximal anchor, test the range of motion (ROM) manually, making sure that full extension is blocked by at least 2° (remember that skin on the upper arm is very mobile).

4. Reapply original anchors to lock down the ends. Spiral up the arm with a cohesive bandage as far as the axilla to prevent skin drag. Secure the end with a strip of tape.

Figure 11.6

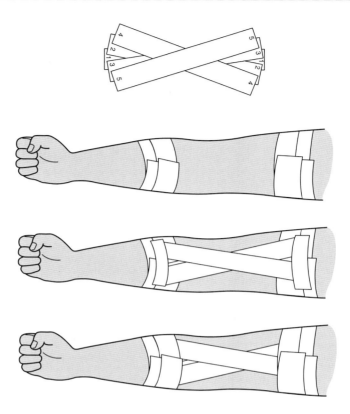

CHECK FUNCTION   Can the patient hold a racket comfortably, and swing
forehand/backhand with confidence?

CONTRAINDICATION   Skin allergy or friable skin.

Tips

The check rein is very useful for blocking ROM at many joints –
wrist (flexion/extension, radial/ulnar deviation), ankle joint,
knee (genu recurvatum).

Prophylactic wrist taping

D. Reese

INDICATION	Prevention of injuries by wrist extension in sport, for example, in gymnastics, strength training and others.
FUNCTION	To reduce wrist extension by applying material over the dorsal aspect of the wrist, without causing circulation restriction and carpal tunnel problems often associated with supporting the wrist.
MATERIALS	2.5/3.75-cm tape, depending on the size of the wrist. A small piece of foam rubber, shaped to cover the palmar aspect of the wrist.
POSITION	Patient standing or sitting while making a fist.
APPLICATION	The patient should be clean, dry and shaved in the area to be taped. Start by having the patient actively make a fist. Place a spongy foam-rubber square on the palmar side of the wrist to protect the tendons (Fig. 11.7).
Anchors	Anchors 1, 2 and 3 should be placed starting approximately 5 cm proximal to the ulnar and radial styloid (Fig. 11.8). Apply the tape so that it conforms to the natural angle of the lower arm and hand junction. Overlap distally approximately one-third of the width of the first anchor. The bottom part of the last anchor should lie forward to the base of the second to fifth metacarpals. Check to see that the anchors do not constrict the ROM.
Support	The support should cover the entire dorsal aspect of the wrist from the styloid processes to the base of the second to fifth metacarpals. The tape is taken back and forth over the area but never circular. The amount is dependent on the amount of support required. Five to six overlaps are common (Fig. 11.9).
Anchor lock	Anchors 1, 2 and 3 should be placed covering the first three (Fig. 11.10).

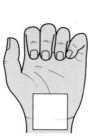

Figure 11.7

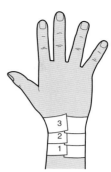

Figure 11.8

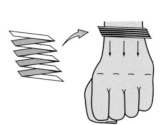

Figure 11.9

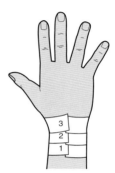

Figure 11.10

CHECK FUNCTION

Is the wrist support adequate for the manoeuvre? If not, adjust by applying more material over the dorsal aspect of the wrist. Check action.

CONTRAINDICATIONS

Circulation problems to the hand can occur if proper application is not followed. This taping is to be used only when the patient is active.

Tips

Best applied directly to the skin dorsally.

Notes

The anchors alone, applied as described above, may be used as a simple wrist taping for strength.

Wrist taping

K.E. Wright

INDICATION	Sprain and strains to the wrist.
FUNCTION	To provide support and stability for the wrist.
MATERIALS	3.8-cm adhesive tape, and 7.5-cm elastic tape.
POSITION	For hyperextension injuries, position wrist in slight flexion and fingers spread apart. For hyperflexion injuries, position wrist in slight extension and fingers spread apart.

APPLICATION

Steps

1. Apply an anchor strip of 3.8-cm adhesive tape around the mid-forearm.

2. Using 7.5-cm elastic tape, cut a strip 30–40 cm in length. In the middle of the tape strip, cut two small holes, approximately 2.5 cm from each side of the tape (Fig. 11.11). With full tension applied to the tape, place the third and fourth phalanges through the cut-outs (Fig. 11.12). Attach the ends of the elastic tape to the mid-forearm anchor (Fig. 11.13).

3. Secure the procedure by applying an anchor of 3.8-cm adhesive tape over the tape ends (Fig. 11.14).

Figure 11.11

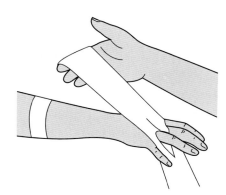

Figure 11.12

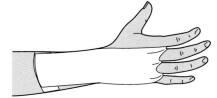

Figure 11.13

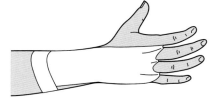

Figure 11.14

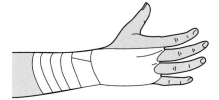

Wrist taping

R. Macdonald

INDICATION	Wrist hyperextension, hyperflexion injury.
FUNCTION	To support and limit ROM.
MATERIALS	Adhesive spray, gauze pad, 3.8-cm and 2.5-cm tape, cohesive bandage.
POSITION	The hand is placed in the open position for anchors, facing operator.
APPLICATION	Spray the hand and wrist. Apply pad to the palmar aspect of the wrist, to protect tendons.

Anchors

1. Using 3.8-cm tape, apply either a diagonal anchor across the hand and around the wrist, or an anchor around the middle of the hand. Apply two anchors around the mid-forearm below muscle bulk (Fig. 11.15). With the hand in a slightly flexed position, measure the distance between the proximal and hand anchors.

Check rein

2. Using 2.0/2.5-cm tape, construct the check rein (fan) on the table (Fig. 11.16), with five or seven strips, overlapping each strip by half.

3. Apply the fan to the hand anchor first and lock in place. Check the ROM of the wrist joint, blocking full extension/flexion. Apply the other end to the forearm anchor. Remember that the skin on the forearm is very mobile.

Lock strips

Apply strips across the ends of the fan to hold in place, then reapply the original anchors (Fig. 11.17). When applying tape: for hyperextension, slightly flex the wrist; for hyperflexion, slightly extend the wrist.

CHECK FUNCTION

Is pronation/supination restricted? Can the patient hold the racket/bat?

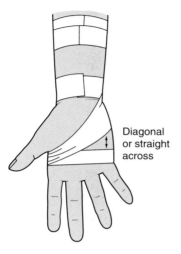

Diagonal or straight across

Figure 11.15

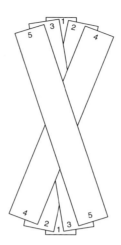

Figure 11.16

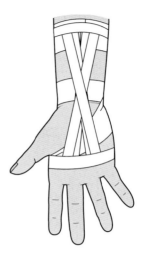

Figure 11.17

Tips

Wrap the hand and wrist with a flesh-coloured cohesive bandage.

Inferior radioulnar joint taping

W.A. Hing and D.A. Reid

INDICATION   Wrist pain, especially with supination or pronation of the wrist. Post-Colles fracture and conditions in which mobilizations with movement (MWMs) are painfree and successful.

FUNCTION   Repositions or corrects a positional fault of the ulna in relation to the radius.

MATERIALS   Spray adhesive or hypoallergenic undertape (Fixomull or Mefix). 38-mm strapping tape.

POSITION   Patient sitting or standing with arm relaxed and wrist in neutral position.

APPLICATION   **Steps**
Taping if a dorsal glide of the ulna on the radius corrects painful movement.

1.   Place tape over palmar surface of the ulna.

2.   Apply and maintain an MWM to the ulna (Fig. 11.18).

3.   In a dorsal direction, wrap tape obliquely across the wrist and around the radius (Fig. 11.19).

4.   Tape will end on the palmar aspect of the wrist, near where the taping began.

5.   Place a second piece of tape on the initial taping to secure.

CHECK FUNCTION   Ensure there is full ROM at the wrist. Assess original painful movements (wrist pronation and supination). Movements should now have painfree full ROM and function.

CONTRAINDICATION   If taping causes changes, or an increase, in pain. Tape should not be left on for >48 h, and should be removed at any hint of skin irritation.

Figure 11.18

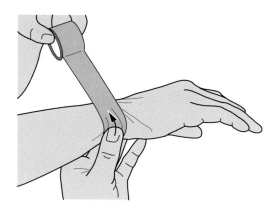

Figure 11.19

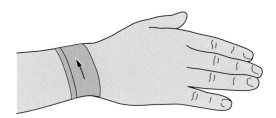

Tips

This procedure is easy to apply with the patient in the correct position, so a family member could be taught to do the taping. This would allow the tape to be removed at night and reapplied in the morning, preventing the risk of an adverse skin reaction.

Contusion to the hand

K.E. Wright

INDICATION	Contusion to the hand.
FUNCTION	To provide protection to the bruised hand.
MATERIALS	2.5-cm and 1.25-cm adhesive tape, 5-cm elastic tape, and felt or foam pad.
POSITION	Hands palmar aspect down and phalanges abducted.
APPLICATION	**Steps**

1. Cut the foam pad before beginning your procedure.

2. Apply an anchor strip of 2.5-cm adhesive tape around the wrist. Start at the ulnar condyle, cross the dorsal aspect of the distal forearm and encircle the wrist (Fig. 11.20). The foam pad is then applied over the affected area of the hand.

3. Apply strips of 1.25-cm tape. Start on the palmar aspect of the anchor strip, cross between the phalanges and end on the dorsal aspect of the anchor strip (Fig. 11.21). Three strips are applied, between the second and third, third and fourth, and fourth and fifth phalanges (Fig. 11.22).

4. Next, apply a strip of 2.5-cm adhesive tape in a figure-of-eight pattern (Fig. 11.23). Begin on the wrist's dorsal aspect near the ulnar condyle; cross diagonally to the second metacarpal, encircling the distal aspect of the second to fifth metacarpals (Fig. 11.24). Continue across the palmar aspect to the fifth metacarpal, crossing diagonally from here to the radial aspect of the wrist and encircle the wrist (Fig. 11.25). Two to three figure-of-eights can be applied.

5. This technique is completed with a second anchor strip of 2.5-cm adhesive tape applied around the wrist. A continuous figure-of-eight strip of 5-cm elastic tape is applied to give additional support (Fig. 11.26).

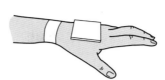

Figure 11.20

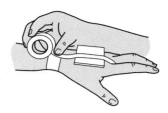

Figure 11.21

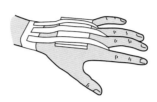

Figure 11.22

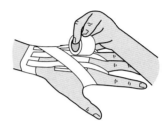

Figure 11.23

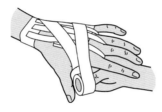

Figure 11.24

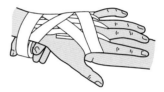

Figure 11.25

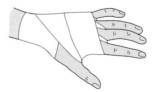

Figure 11.26

Palm protective taping (the Russell web)

C. Armstrong

INDICATION	Unconditioned/uncalloused palms in gymnastics.

FUNCTION	• to act as a layer of protection over the skin on the palm of the hand. • To help the patient maintain a grip on gymnastic apparatus.

MATERIALS	Adhesive spray, lubricant, 10/7.5-cm stretch tape, 3.75-cm tape.

POSITION	The patient is standing with the arm held forwards and palm up.

APPLICATION

1. Shave the wrist.

2. Lubricate the web space between the fingers and apply gauze (Fig. 11.27).

3. Apply adhesive spray to the hand, including the wrist.

4. Using a length of 10-cm stretch tape that stretches to twice the length of the hand, attach the tape to the base of the hand so that the hand is in the middle of the length of tape (Fig. 11.28).

5. Starting at the finger-end of the tape, make four longitudinal cuts into the tape so that, when stretched, the tape strands fit between the fingers but the unsplit portion covers the palm (Fig. 11.29a).

6. Bring these taut strips up from the palmar aspect of the hand to go on the outside of the index finger on the one side and the little finger on the other. The middle strips come up into the web spaces between each of the fingers. These strips should run down the back of the hand, across the wrist, ending on the back of the distal forearm at the wrist (Fig. 11.29b).

Figure 11.27

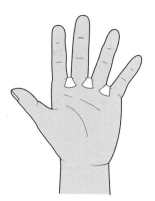

Figure 11.28

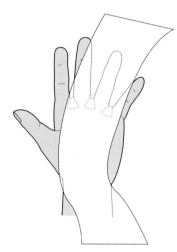

Figure 11.29

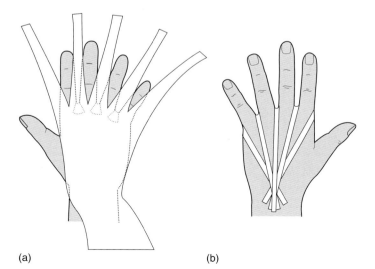

(a)   (b)

7. Then, going to the wrist end of the length of tape, cut it down the middle, allowing the cut to correspond to the distal wrist crease. The two strips should be stretched and run around the wrist, anchoring the strands that come along the dorsum of the hand to the wrist (Fig. 11.30a).

8. Cover the wrist strips with 3.75-cm tape (Fig. 11.30b).

CHECK FUNCTION

- The patient should be able to flex and extend the wrist without undue discomfort from the tape cutting into the web space between the fingers.

- The tape should be sufficiently taut not to allow any bunching.

CONTRAINDICATIONS

None.

Tips

On a smaller hand, one might be well-advised to use 7.5-cm rather than 10-cm stretch tape.

Figure 11.30

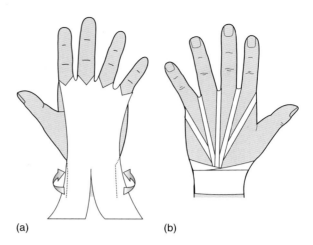

(a)   (b)

Protection of the metacarpophalangeal joints for boxers

R. Macdonald

INDICATION

To protect the metacarpophalangeal joints for boxers when training, and in combat sports.

FUNCTION

- to maintain the protective padding in place.
- to leave the palm free for gripping in martial arts.

MATERIALS

2.5- and 5-cm stretch tape, adhesive spray, padding/PPT/Poron or rubber.

APPLICATION

Steps

1. Spray the dorsum of the hand and wrist. Cut a protective pad to fit over the four metacarpophalangeal joints. Stick the pad in place and anchor it with 5-cm stretch tape. Apply 5-cm stretch tape anchor around the wrist (Fig. 11.31).

2. Using 2.5-cm stretch tape, cut four strips long enough to encircle each finger, and anchor on the proximal end of the wrist anchor.

3. The centre of the first strip is placed around the index finger. Cross the two ends over the metacarpophalangeal joint. One winds over the metacarpal of the thumb to attach to the anterior aspect of the wrist anchor. The other end is attached to the wrist anchor, on the dorsum (Fig. 11.32).

4. Repeat this on the middle and ring fingers. Finger 5 is the same as the index finger, with one strip winding around to the palmar aspect of the wrist anchor (Fig. 11.33).

Lock strips

Reapply the wrist anchor and close off with the tape (Fig. 11.34).

Notes

The pad may be bevelled to overlay the web of the fingers or lubricated gauze pads may be applied between the fingers.

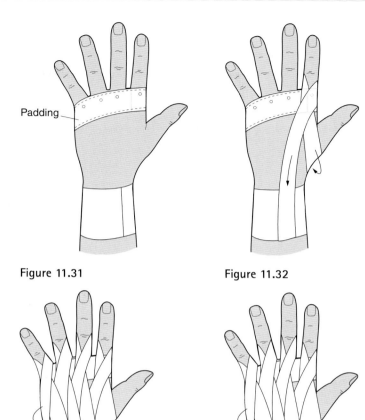

Padding

Figure 11.31   Figure 11.32

Figure 11.33   Figure 11.34

CHECK FUNCTION   Can the athlete make a fist without discomfort? Is the pad in the right position for full protection?

CONTRAINDICATIONS   None.

Tips

Apply adhesive spray directly to the pad. Let it get tacky before sticking it to the metacarpophalangeal joints. If secure, the anchor may not be necessary.

Chapter **12**

Fingers and thumb

CHAPTER CONTENTS

Sprained fingers – buddy system   208
Single-finger taping   210
Finger joint support   212
Climber's finger injury   214

Prophylactic thumb taping   216
Simple thumb check-rein figure-of-eight
   method   220
Thumb spica taping   222

Sprained fingers – buddy system

R. Macdonald

INDICATION	Minor trauma to finger on the field of play, ball hitting the extended finger, jammed finger.
FUNCTION	To protect and support the finger by taping it to its neighbour (functional splint).
MATERIALS	Foam or felt padding, 2.5-cm tape.
POSITION	Standing, facing the operator with hand outstretched, and fingers held slightly apart.
APPLICATION	**Steps**

1. Place a strip of felt, foam or cotton wool between the injured finger and the adjacent fingers.
2. Apply strips of tape around the proximal and middle phalanges, with the closures on the dorsal aspect.
3. Do not cover the joint lines with tape.
4. Two or three fingers may be taped together, depending on the sport (Fig. 12.1).

CHECK FUNCTION	Can the patient hold equipment, grasp, throw and catch?
CONTRAINDICATION	Suspected fracture, ligament tear, or tendon avulsion.

Tips

Tape may be ripped down the centre for a small finger.

Figure 12.1

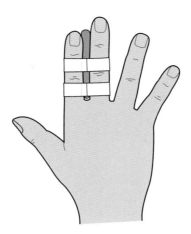

Single–finger taping

J. O'Neill

FUNCTION	To help support the collateral ligaments of the fingers.
MATERIALS	Tape adherent, 1.25-cm porous tape.
POSITION	The athlete's injured finger is extended in a relaxed position.
APPLICATION	This technique is similar to taping of collateral ligament sprain of a knee.

1. Apply tape adherent.

2. Apply a 1.25-cm anchor strip around the middle and proximal phalanx (Fig. 12.2).

3. Eight strips of 1.25-cm tape approximately 5–8 cm long are precut and then applied as indicated in Figure 12.3.

4. Place a 2.5-cm. strip to cover tape around the middle and proximal phalanx (Fig. 12.4).

5. Finally, 'buddy tape' the injured finger to the adjacent finger to aid in support (Fig. 12.5).

CHECK FUNCTION	Be watchful of overtightness of the tape.

Tips

When taping fingers, place in about 15° of flexion. This will allow the athlete to feel more comfortable.

Figure 12.2

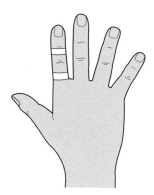

Figure 12.3

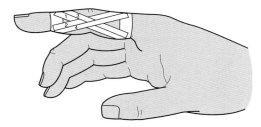

Figure 12.4

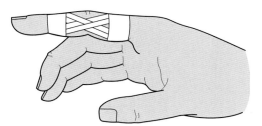

Figure 12.5

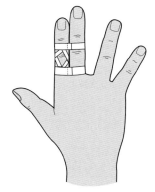

Finger joint support

R. Macdonald

INDICATION	Collateral ligament sprain.
FUNCTION	To support the joint in a functional position, allowing flexion and extension of the digits.
MATERIALS	2.5-cm tape, which may be ripped down the centre for a small finger.
POSITION	Facing the operator, hand in prone position with the fingers held apart.

APPLICATION

Steps

1. Cover the finger nail with a small piece of tape, sticky sides folded together by two-thirds. Stick on just above the nail (Fig. 12.6).

2. Measure the finger from the metacarpophalangeal joint to the finger tip, and rip four strips.

3. Lay one strip diagonally across the proximal interphalangeal joint and wrap the ends around the proximal and distal phalanges (Fig. 12.6).

4. Repeat on the other side of the joint.

5. Apply these same strips twice more, making sure that the tape does not cover the joint line (Fig. 12.7).

6. Secure the tape with proximal and distal anchors.

CHECK FUNCTION	Can the patient use the finger normally?
CONTRAINDICATION	Suspected fracture, joint disruption or tendon avulsion.

Figure 12.6

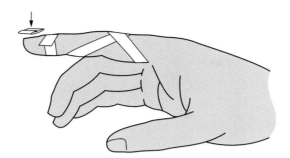

Figure 12.7

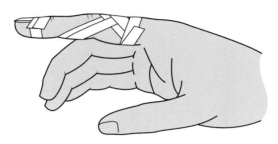

 Tips

Cover with a finger stall or cohesive bandage if going in water.
A glove may be worn with this technique.

Climber's finger injury

R. Macdonald

INDICATION	Finger flexor tendon strain in climbers, usually the fourth or ring finger.
FUNCTION	Stabilizes the finger in a flexed position and limits extension of the proximal interphalangeal joint.
MATERIALS	2.5-cm rigid tape, 2.5-cm adhesive bandage.
POSITION	Sitting with the supinated forearm resting on a table and hand over the edge, with the finger flexed.

APPLICATION

Steps

1. Take about a 15-cm length of tape.
2. Split one end and wrap around the proximal phalanx from the palmar aspect; apply an anchor with the closure on the dorsal aspect.
3. Roll the tape between thumb and index finger to form a rope (Fig. 12.8).
4. Split the other end of the tape and wrap around the middle or distal phalanx (depending on which tendon is strained) to maintain the finger in the flexed position (Fig. 12.9).
5. Place another anchor around the distal phalanx with closure on the dorsal aspect.
6. Wrap the finger with cohesive bandage.

CHECK FUNCTION	Check that the phalanx is held in the flexed position and is stable. Check circulation.
CONTRAINDICATION	Do not place tape on the nail as it may damage the nail bed on removal.

Figure 12.8

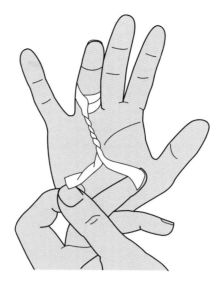

Figure 12.9

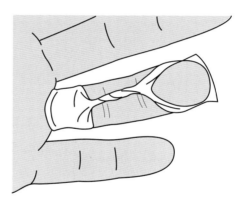

 Tips

Prior to taping, cover the nail with a small piece of tape folded sticky sides together, with a little bit of the adhesive mass free to stick on the finger proximal to the nail.

Prophylactic thumb taping

D. Reese

INDICATION
Prevention of injuries caused by hyperextension of the thumb in sports, for example, ice hockey, European handball, skiing, soccer goalkeepers.

FUNCTION
To prevent hyperextension of the thumb and further damage to the volar ligament without inhibiting any other of the vital functions of the thumb. Its simplicity allows the athlete to regulate the tension at any time for better function.

MATERIALS
2.5/1.25-cm tape stripped (less than the width of the thumb). A small piece of foam rubber shaped to cover the palmar aspect of the wrist.

POSITION
The patient is standing or sitting.

APPLICATION
The hand should be clean, dry and shaved in the area to be taped. Start by having the patient actively make a fist. Place a spongy foam-rubber square on the palmar side of the wrist to protect the wrist tendons (Fig. 12.10).

Anchors
Anchors 1 and 2 should be placed starting approximately 5 cm proximal to the ulnar and radial styloid. Apply the tape so that it conforms to the natural angle of the lower arm and hand junction. Overlap distally approximately one-third of the width of the first anchor. Check to see that the anchors do not constrict the range of motion (Fig. 12.11).

Figure 12.10

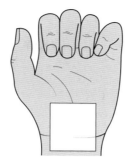

Figure 12.11

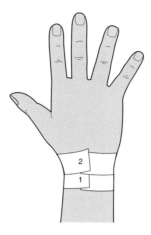

Support

Place two strips 60 cm in length that are a little less than the width of the thumb on top of each other. Open the hand and start the support at the base of the first phalanx on the dorsal side of the hand. Pull the tape through the middle line of the thumb over the thumb nail and over the volar ligament towards the ulnar styloid on the palmar side of the hand (Figs 12.12 and 12.13). Wrap the rest of the support around the wrist (Fig. 12.14).

Lock strip

Lock a small strip around the second phalanx of the thumb as well as a couple of strips on top of each other over the base of the first phalanx (Fig. 12.15).

CHECK FUNCTION

Allow the patient to decide the tension and restriction of the tape that will be used in the activity. Have on hand the equipment or ball for final adjustment.

CONTRAINDICATION

Hypermobility in hyperextension of the thumb.

Tips

Inform the patient that adjustments may be made during the activity by pulling up the end of the tape and reapplying new tension around the wrist.

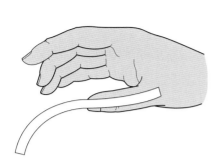

Figure 12.12

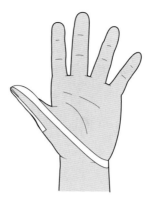

Figure 12.13

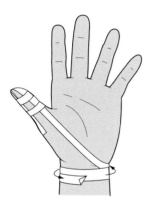

Figure 12.14

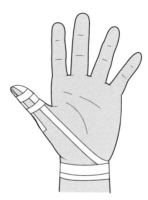

Figure 12.15

Simple thumb check-rein figure-of-eight method

R. Macdonald

INDICATION   Thumb hyperextension.

FUNCTION   To stabilize the joint and restrict extension and abduction of the thumb.

MATERIALS   2.5-cm or 1.25-cm tape.

POSITION   The hand is held in a functional position. (Face the operator to shake hands.)

APPLICATION   Start on the dorsal aspect of the proximal aspect of the thumb. Draw tape around the thumb towards the palm, then through the web, twisting the tape. Continue over the dorsal aspect of the hand, moulding the tape to the skin, then around and across the palmar surface to web moulding tape to the palm.
Draw the thumb towards the palm into a functional position and attach the tape to the starting point (do not wind the end around the thumb) (Fig. 12.16).
Apply this check rein over any thumb tape job.

Notes

- to control extension – apply tension towards the palmar surface.
- to control abduction – apply tension towards the dorsal surface.

Figure 12.16

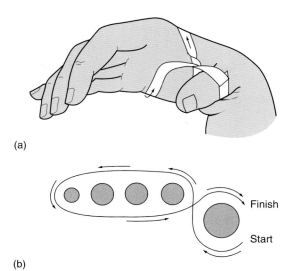

(a)

Finish

Start

(b)

Tips

Use adhesive spray on the palm of the hand for better
adhesion, and mould adhesive mass to the palm.
Check circulation by pressing the thumb nail.

Thumb spica taping

K.E. Wright

INDICATION	Thumb sprain.
FUNCTION	To provide support and stability for the first metacarpophalangeal joint of the hand.
MATERIAL	2.5-cm adhesive tape.
POSITION	Hand in palm-down position, with thumb slightly flexed and phalanges adducted.
APPLICATION	**Steps**

1. Apply an anchor strip of adhesive tape around the wrist (Fig. 12.17). Start at the ulnar condyle, cross the dorsal aspect of the distal forearm and encircle the wrist.

2. Apply the first of three support strips for the first metacarpophalangeal joint (Fig. 12.18). Starting at the ulnar condyle, cross the dorsum of the hand, cover the lateral joint line, encircle the thumb, proceed across the palmar aspect of the hand and finish at the ulnar condyle (Fig. 12.19).

3. Repeat step 2 twice (Fig. 12.20).

4. To help hold this procedure in place, apply a final anchor strip around the wrist (Fig. 12.21).

Figure 12.17

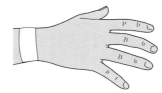

Figure 12.18

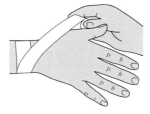

Figure 12.19

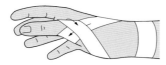

Figure 12.20

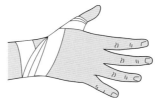

Figure 12.21

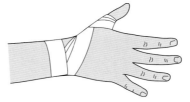

Chapter **13**

Stretch tape – many uses

R. Macdonald

One is sometimes in a position when there is a limited supply of tape available for use. One strip of tape may be adapted for many uses and, in many cases, lends itself to self-application. The following are some ideas for using a length of stretch tape with its ends cut or torn into four tails (Fig. 13.1). The adhesive mass on the uncut centre portion may be covered with another piece, sticky sides together, or reinforced with a piece of rigid tape for more strength. Applying talcum powder to the adhesive side eliminates the sticky mass from the tape (Figs 13.2–13.7).

Figure 13.1 7.5-/10-cm stretch tape.

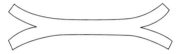

Figure 13.2 Achilles tendon support.

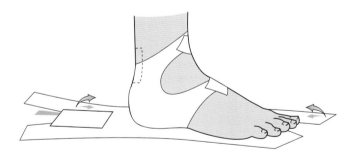

Figure 13.3 (a) and (b) 7.5-/10-cm stretch tape used for patellar support.

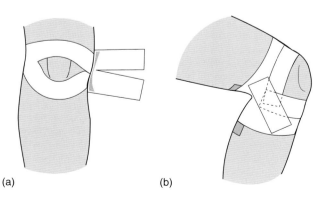

(a) (b)

Figure 13.4 Achilles tendon support.

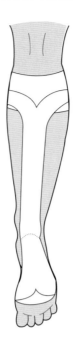

Figure 13.5 Tape used to support dorsiflexors (dropped foot).

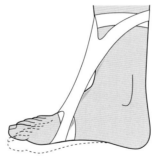

Figure 13.6 (a) and (b) To block full extension of the elbow.

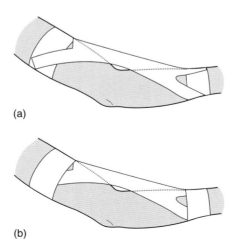

(a)

(b)

Figure 13.7   Tape used to support extensor tendons (dropped wrist).

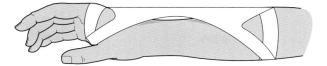

Chapter 14

Spicas and triangular bandages

R. Macdonald

The spica or figure-of-eight bandage is very useful for a variety of conditions and can often be self-applied. In some situations, the spica is more appropriate than tape and is often used as a first-aid measure to protect the injured structure, to restrict range of motion and to minimize swelling and bleeding (Figs 14.1–14.6). Elastic stretch tape or any type of non-adhesive bandage may be used. If the support is to be removed for the application of cold or heat or therapeutic exercise, then a bandage is more appropriate as it may be used many times and is less costly. The spica must be applied firmly but not too tightly, each strip overlapping the previous one

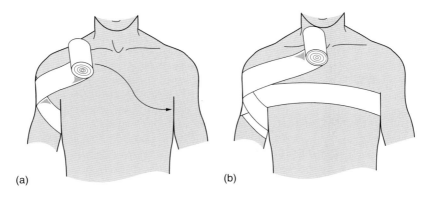

(a)　　　　　　　　　　　　　(b)

Figure 14.1　(a) and (b)
Shoulder spica.

Figure 14.2 (a) and (b) Bandage to support a dislocation of the acromioclavicular and/or shoulder joint.

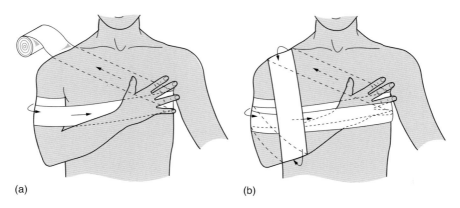

(a)   (b)

Figure 14.3 (a) and (b) Ankle and foot spica.

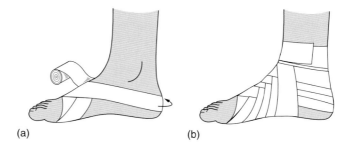

(a)   (b)

Figure 14.4 (a–d) Ankle wrap.

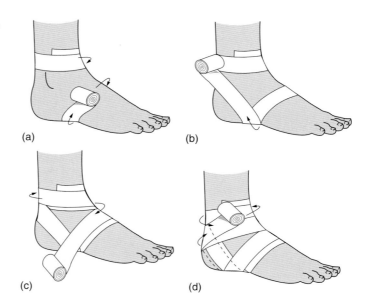

(a)   (b)

(c)   (d)

Figure 14.5 (a–c) Elastic groin support.

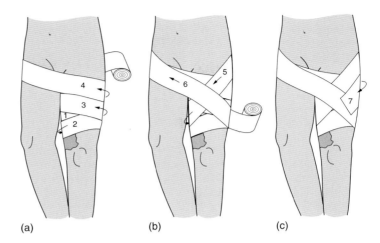

(a) (b) (c)

Figure 14.6 (a) and (b) Thumb spicas.

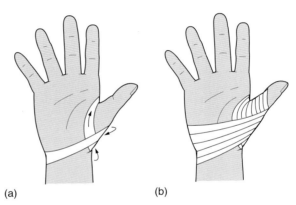

(a) (b)

by half. A cold, wet spica is ideal for an acute injury. After application, check circulation and neural transmission.

Figure 14.7 A sling for a fractured collarbone. Reproduced by kind permission of St John Ambulance. © Copyright 2003.

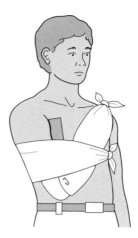

Figure 14.8 (a–c) Folding a triangular bandage. Reproduced by kind permission of St John Ambulance. © Copyright 2003.

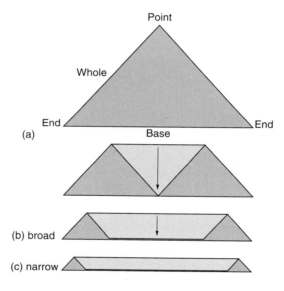

Figure 14.9   Preparing an arm sling. Reproduced by kind permission of St John Ambulance. © Copyright 2003.

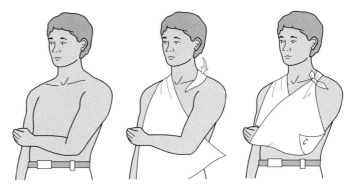

Figure 14.10   Preparing an elevation sling. Reproduced by kind permission of St John Ambulance. © Copyright 2003.

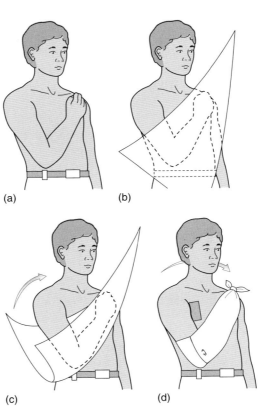

(a)   (b)

(c)   (d)

Glossary

Abduction movement	away from the midline of the body
Achilles tendon	tendon behind heel
Acromioclavicular joint	AC joint
Adduction movement	towards the midline of the body
Adhesive mass	sticky backing on tape
Anterior	front
Anterior cruciate	ligament within the knee joint, limits anterior movement of tibia on femur
Assess	evaluate
Biceps	muscle on front of upper arm
Calcaneum	heel bone
Check rein	reinforced tape to restrict movement
Cohesive bandage	rubberized, sticks to itself and not to the skin
Condyle	bony end of thigh bone
Contract	tense
Contusion	bruise
Digit	finger/toe
Distal	area away from centre of body or furthest attachment
Dorsal	back (e.g. of hand)
Extension	to straighten
Extensor tendons	on front of ankle joint
Femur	thigh bone
Flexion	to bend
Friction	rubbing
Hamstring	muscle at back of thigh
Hyperextend	to extend beyond the normal
Hypoallergenic	will not cause reaction on sensitive skin
Inferior	below
Innominate bones	flat bones that form pelvic girdle
Inversion	turning in, e.g. ankle sprain
Kinesiology	study of motion of human body
Lateral	side away from the body, outside
Ligaments	taut bands of tissue which bind bones together
Longitudinal arch	from heel to toes on undersurface of foot
Malleolus	ankle bone
Medial	side closest to the body, inside

Palmar	front (e.g. of hand)
Patella	knee cap
Pes cavus	foot with high rigid arch
Pes planus	foot with flat longitudinal arch
Peritenonitis	inflammation of the tendon sheath
Plantar fascia	tough bands of tissue on sole of foot
Plantar fasciitis	inflammation at origin of plantar fascia (near heel)
Plantarflex	toes and foot pointed downwards, towards floor
Popliteal fossa	space behind knee
Posterior	behind, rear
Pronate	turn palm-down
Pronated feet	flat feet
Prone	lying face-down
Proprioception	awareness of body position, perception of movement and change of direction
Proximal	close to centre of body or nearest attachment
Quadriceps	muscles at front of thigh
Rehabilitate	to treat and restore to normal health
Rotator cuff	stabilizing muscles for the shoulder
Spica	figure-of-eight bandage technique
Sprain	overstretching or tearing of a ligament
Strain	overstretching or tearing of a muscle
Superior	above
Supinate	turn palm-up
Supine	lying on the back, facing upward
Tendinosis	degeneration in the tendon itself
Thenar eminence	muscular area of thumb on palm of hand (intrinsic muscles)
Tibia	shin bone
Tibial tubercle	tibial attachment for the patellar tendon
Transverse arch	from medial to lateral
Valgus	distal bone/part pointing away from the midline of body, knock knees
Varus	distal part/bone pointing toward the midline of the body, bow legs

Index

A

Achilles tendinitis, 36, 96
Achilles tendinopathy, 94–95
Achilles tendon
  referred pain, 84
  support, 100–103, 225, 226
    rear foot stabilization, 102–103
    self-application, 98–99
    simple method, 100–101
Acromioclavicular joint
  dislocation, 230
  strap, 164–165
  subluxation, 162–163
  taping, 166–169
    modified for gleno-humeral instabilities, 168, 169
    for sport using stretch tape, 170–173
Activity, return to, 5
Adhesive capsulitis, 176
Adhesive spray, 8
Allingham's strap, 178–179
Anchors, 7
Ankle, 87–113
  braces, 11
  closed basketweave taping, 108–109
  controlling oedema, 9–10
  dorsiflexion and rear foot motion control, 96–97
  functional instability, 10
  inferior tibiofibular joint, 92–93
  injury prevention, 11
  literature update, 9–11
  mechanical instability, 10
  preventive taping to lateral aspect, 104–107
  prewrap, 11
  spica, 230
  taping technique, 11
  wrap, 230
  see also Achilles tendon
Ankle sprain
  acute, 90–91
    field wrap, 88–89

  closed basketweave taping, 108–109
  heel locks for closed basketweave, 110–111
  ligament and tendon support after, 82–83
  prevention of recurrent, 11
  subtalar instabilities after, 96
Anterior cruciate ligament (ACL)
  elongation, 136
  sprain, 132–133
  support, 130–131
Anterior talofibular ligament sprain, 104
Antipronation taping, 70–71
Apical crescent, 45
Apical pads, 44–45
Application, tape, 6–7
Arm elevation sling, 233
Arm sling, 233

B

Back and leg pain, chronic low, 21–23, 148–149
Back pain, lumbar, 142–143
Bandage scissors, 8
Board lasted shoe, 54
Boxers, metacarpophalangeal joint protection, 204–205
Buddy system, sprained fingers, 208–209
Buttock, unloading, 21, 22

C

Calcaneofibular ligament sprain, 104
Calcaneum
  mobilization with movement (MWM), 80
  motion control, 84–85
Check-rein figure-of-eight method, thumb, 220–221
Check reins, 7
  elbow, 188, 189

Chopart's joint (metatarsus equinus), 51, 52
Clavicle, fractured, 232
Climber's finger injury, 214–215
Cloth wrap, 8
Cohesive bandages, 4–5, 8
Collarbone, fractured, 232
Collateral ligaments of fingers
  single-finger taping to support, 210–211
  sprains, 212–213
Colles fracture, post, 196
Combination lasted shoe, 54–55
Crystal Palace wrap, 124–125
Cuboid subluxation in dancers, 78–79
Curved lasted shoe, 54

D

D pad, 32–34
Dancers, cuboid subluxation, 78–79
Dehesive spray, 8
Diamond wrap, 126–127
Digits *see* Fingers; Toes
Dorsal crescent pad, foot, 38–40
Dorsal pads, foot, 38–40
Dorsiflexion, ankle, and rear foot motion control, 96–97
Dorsiflexors, foot, support, 226
Dumbbell pad, 43–44
Dye's model of tissue homeostasis of joint, 16

E

Elastic adhesive tape *see* Stretch adhesive tape
Elastic bandage, 8
Elbow, 184–189
  extension, blocking, 226
  hyperextension sprain, 188–189
  impingement, 188
  tennis, 184–187

Equinus foot, 51–52
   compensated, 52
   heel pads, 36
   metatarsus, 51
   partially compensated, 51–52
   talipes, 51
Extensor tendons of wrist,
      support, 227

F

Fat pad, infrapatellar
   irritation, 18, 19–20, 122
   unloading, 118–119, 122–123
Field, taping player on, 5
Field wrap, acute ankle sprain,
      88–89
Figure-of-eight bandages
      see Spicas
Figure-of-eight wrap for knee,
      continuous, 134–135
Fingers, 208–215
   climber's injury, 214–215
   joint support, 212–213
   single-finger taping, 210–211
   sprained, buddy system,
      208–209
First metatarsophalangeal (MTP)
      joint
   sprain, 62, 64
   valgus strain, 66–67
Flexor hallucis longus tendon
      irritation, 82
Flexor tendon strains, finger,
      in climbers, 214–215
Foot, 61–85
   antipronation taping, 70–71
   calcaneal motion control, 84–85
   cuboid subluxation in dancers,
      78–79
   dorsiflexors, support, 226
   dropped, 226
   first-aid padding, 29–45
   great toe taping, 64–65
   hallux valgus, 66–67
   heel pain, 80–81
   hyperpronation, 70
   ideal relationship, 46
   ligament and tendon support,
      82–83
   medial arch support, 76–77
   plantar fasciitis support, 72–73
   plantar fasciitis taping, 74–75
   spica, 230
   support, 68–69
   turf toe strap, 62–63
   types, 45–53
Footwear, 53–57
   lacing methods, 55–57
   sports, 53–55
Forefoot valgus, 50–51
   flexible, 50–51
   rigid, 50

Forefoot varus, 48–50
   fully compensated, 49–50
   partially compensated, 49
   uncompensated, 49
Frontal plane pelvic stability,
      144–145

G

Gauze squares, 7
Gibney strips, 7
Gleno-humeral joint instability
   acromioclavicular joint taping
      adapted for, 167, 168
   anterior, 174–175
   multidirectional, 24, 180–181
Great toe
   joint see First metatarso-
      phalangeal (MTP) joint
   taping, 64–65
Groin support, elastic, 231
Guidelines, taping, 5–6

H

Hallux valgus, 66–67
Hand, 198–205
   contusion, 198–199
   metacarpophalangeal joint
      protection for boxers,
      204–205
   palm protective taping, 200–203
Heel bumps, 36
Heel locks, 7, 110–111
Heel pad, 34–36
Heel pain, 80–81
Heel wedges, 36–38
   lateral, 37
   medial, 36, 37
Hinton–Boswell method, ankle
      taping, 11
Horizontal strips, 7
Horseshoe pad, 41–42
Humeral head
   excessive translation, 23
   relocation, 23–24, 176–177
Hypoallergenic tapes, 4

I

Iliotibial band (ITB) friction
      syndrome, 144
Impingement
   elbow, 188
   shoulder, 23, 176, 178–179
Inferior radioulnar joint taping,
      196–197
Inferior tibiofibular joint, 92–93
Inflammation, minimizing
      aggravation, 16–17

Infrapatellar fat pad see Fat pad,
      infrapatellar
Interdigital pads, 42–43

J

Joint
   Dye's model of tissue
      homeostasis, 16
   neutral zone, 16
   stability, 15–16
Jumper's knee, 120, 124

K

Knee, 115–139
   anterior cruciate taping,
      132–133
   arthroscopy, post, 122
   continuous figure-of-eight
      wrap, 134–135
   hyperextended, 122
   jumper's, 120, 124
   lateral collateral ligament
      sprain, 128–129
   pain, 116–117
      posterolateral, 112
      retropatellar, 120, 124
      see also Patellofemoral
         pain
   patellar tendinosis, 118–119
   runner's, 144
   sprains, 134–135
   stabilization, 128–131
   support, 120–121
      Crystal Palace wrap,
         124–125
      diamond wrap, 126–127
      variation, 130–131
   unstable, 136–139

L

Lacing, shoe, 55–57
   dorsal relief, 57
   independent, 57
   secure rearfoot, 56
   single-lace cross, 55
   square-box, 55
   variable-width, 56
Lateral collateral ligament sprain,
      128–129
Lateral epicondylosis (tennis
      elbow), 184–185
   simple technique, 186–187
Leg, 87–113
Leg-length discrepancy, 52–53
Ligament and tendon support,
      foot, 82–83
Lock strips, 7

Low-back and leg pain, chronic, 21–23, 148–149
Low-back pain, 142–143
Lumbar dysfunction and pain, 142–143
Lumbar spine, 141–149
    frontal plane pelvic stability, 144–145
    stabilizing unstable segments, 23
    taping, 142–143

M

Medial arch support, 76–77
Medial collateral ligament sprain, 188
Metacarpophalangeal joint protection for boxers, 204–205
Metatarsal shaft pad, 32
Metatarsus equinus, 51, 52
Mylanta, 95, 119

N

Nails, finger, 214, 215
Neck pain, 152
Neural tissue, unloading, 21–23
Non-stretch adhesive tape, 4

O

Osgood–Schlatter's disease, 118, 124

P

Padding, 7
    foot, 29–45
Pain, 15–27
    effect of tape, 17–18
    unloading principle, 16–17
    see also specific pain syndromes
Palm protective taping, 200–203
Patellar taping, 18, 225
    case study, 19–20
    effect on pain, 17–18
    effect on patellar position, 17
    literature update, 11–12
Patellar tendinitis (tendinosis), 18, 118–119, 136
Patellofemoral dysfunction, 120
Patellofemoral pain (syndrome), 12, 18–20, 116–117
    foot support, 68
    frontal plane pelvic stability, 144
    inferior, 122

patellar taping see Patellar taping
    specific VMO training, 20
Pelvic stability, frontal plane, 144–145
Pelvic tilt, excessive lateral horizontal, 144
Peroneal weakness, reflex, 84
Peroneus tendon strain, 104
Petroleum jelly, 8
Piriformis syndrome, 144
Plantar cover pads, 31–32
Plantar fasciitis, 36, 68
    chronic, 80
    support, 72–73
    taping, 74–75
Plantar metatarsal pads (PMPs), 29–31
Posterior cruciate ligament (PCL), elongation, 136
Posterior tibiotalar ligament pain, 82
Prewrap, ankle taping with, 11
Principles, taping, 5
Proprioception
    functional ankle instability and, 10
    patellar taping and, 12
Prowrap, 7

Q

Quadriceps
    strengthening, patellofemoral pain, 20
    torque, patellar taping and, 17–18

R

Radioulnar joint, inferior, 196–197
Rearfoot
    motion control, 96–97
    stabilization, Achilles tendon support with, 102–103
    valgus, 47–48
    varus, 45–47
        compensated, 47
        partially compensated, 46–47
        uncompensated, 46
Reinforcing strips, 7
Removal, tape, 7
Return to activity, 5
Rigney's strap, 174–175
Role of taping, 3–4
Rose's bar, 36
Rotator cuff
    tears, 176
    tendinitis, 23
Runner's knee, 144
Russell web, 200–203

S

Sacroiliac joint (SIJ)
    dysfunction, 146–147
    instability, 144
Scapula
    control (Watson's strap), 158–159
    retraction, 160
    winging, 156–157
Scissors, bandage, 8
Semicurved lasted shoe, 54
Shaeffer's joint (metatarsus equinus), 51, 52
Shaft pad, 32
Shin splints, 68
Shoes see Footwear
Shoulder, 161–182
    acromioclavicular joint see Acromioclavicular joint
    Allingham's strap, 178–179
    anterior instability, 174–175
    dislocation, 230
    impingement, 23, 176, 178–179
    multidirectional instability, 24, 180–181
    overactive upper trapezius, 182
    pain, 23–24
    relocation of humeral head, 23–24, 176–177
    spica, 229
Silicone putty, dorsal toe protection, 40
Single-finger taping, 210–211
Sinus tarsi pain, 84
Slip lasted shoe, 54
Spicas (figure-of-eight bandages), 229–231
    thumb, 222–223, 231
Sports footwear, 53–55
Stirrups, 7
Storage, tape, 7
Straight lasted shoe, 53, 54
Straight-leg raise (SLR), 146
Stretch adhesive tape, 4
    multiple uses, 225–227
Subtalar joint
    dysfunction, 80
    instabilities, 96
Superior tibiofibular joint, 112–113
Support strips, 7

T

Talcum powder, 8
Talipes equinus, 51
Tape
    application, 6–7
    handling technique, 4–5
    non-stretch adhesive, 4
    products, 4–5
    removal, 7

Tape (*contd*)
  storage, 7
  stretch *see* Stretch adhesive tape
Tape cutter, 8
Tape remover, 8
Taping
  guidelines, 5–6
  principles, 5
  products, 7–8
  role, 3–4
  terms, 7–8
Tennis elbow, 184–185
  simple technique, 186–187
Tensor, 8
Terms, taping, 7–8
Thoracic facet sprain, 154
Thoracic pain and posture
    correction, 152
Thoracic spine, 151–160
  taping, 152–153
  unload, 154–155
Thumb, 216–223
  check-rein figure-of-eight
      method, 220–221
  hyperextension injuries, 216,
      220
  prophylactic taping, 216–219
  spica taping, 222–223, 231
  sprains, 222
Tibial rotation taping, 116–117
Tibialis posterior tenoperiostitis,
    68

Toes
  interdigital pads, 42–43
  props/splints, 40–41
  see also Great toe
Trapezius, overactive upper, 182
Trendelenburg sign, 144
Triangular bandages, 232–233
Trochanteric bursitis, 144
Tubular bandage, 8
Turf toe (first MTP joint sprain),
    62, 64
  strap, 62–63

U

Underwrap, 7
Unloading
  neural tissue, 21–23
  painful structures, 16–17

V

Valgus
  forefoot, 50–51
  rearfoot, 47–48
Valgus filler pad, 32–33
Varus
  forefoot, 48–50
  rearfoot *see under* Rearfoot

Vastus lateralis (VL)
  inhibition by taping, 20, 21
  magnitude of activation, 18
  timing of activation, 17, 20
Vastus medialis oblique (VMO)
  magnitude of activation, 18
  specific training, 20
  timing of activation, 17, 20
Vleeming test, 146

W

Waterproof tape, 4
Watson's strap, 158–159
Wedges, heel, 36–38
Wrapping products, 4–5
Wrist, 190–197
  dropped, 227
  extension, reduction, 190
  extensor tendon support, 227
  hyperextension injuries, 192,
      194
  hyperflexion injuries, 192, 194
  inferior radioulnar joint
      taping, 196–197
  pain, 196
  prophylactic taping, 190–191
  taping, 192–195